Pharmacy Law Q&A Prep

Kentucky MPJE®

- ☑ 100 KENTUCKY LAW QUESTIONS
- ☑ 100 FEDERAL LAW QUESTIONS

PHARMACY TESTING SOLUTIONS   2022 EDITION

ISBN: 979-8-4076-6823-7

Table of Contents

Introduction

The Multistate Pharmacy Jurisprudence Examination, or MPJE, is the pharmacy law exam created by the National Association of Boards of Pharmacy. It is designed to test your knowledge and competency of pharmacy law. The exam consists of 120 federal and state-specific questions that cover three content areas: pharmacy practice (83% of the questions); licensure, registration, certification, and operational requirements (15% of the questions); and general regulatory processes (2% of the questions).

This book will help you prepare for federal and state questions from all content areas. The first section includes 100 questions on federal pharmacy law. The second section includes 100 questions on Kentucky state pharmacy law. At the back of the book is an answer index with detailed explanations for each question. When taking the MPJE, it is important to choose the most strict answer if there are differences between federal and state laws (unless otherwise instructed to answer specifically federal or state law).

When preparing for the MPJE, remove all distractions, read each question carefully, and try not to refer to any resources. The actual exam is 2½ hours, so you might find it helpful to time yourself to ensure you are not taking too much (or too little) time on each question.

Make sure to spread out your study time as well; cramming the night before an exam is proven to result in low retention and difficulty focusing during the test. Study gradually over time and test your competency and timing using this book.

On the day of the exam, make sure you are well rested, you eat a substantial breakfast, and you leave for the testing center early, so that you will arrive at least 30 minutes before the exam starts. Good luck on the MPJE, and happy studying!

Federal MPJE Practice Questions

1. What was the first law to prohibit the distribution of food and drugs that were misbranded or adulterated?
    a. Food, Drug and Cosmetic Act
    b. Pure Food and Drug Act
    c. Prescription Drug Marketing Act
    d. Durham-Humphrey Amendment
    e. Kefauver-Harris Amendment

2. What is the system that can be used as an electronic substitute for DEA Form 222 when ordering Schedule II controlled substances?
    a. Controlled Online Ordering System
    b. Online Opioid Ordering System
    c. Controlled Substance Ordering System
    d. Federal Controlled Substance Ordering System
    e. Scheduled Substance Ordering System

3. What agency is responsible for the federal Controlled Substances Act (CSA)?
    a. Federal Bureau of Investigation (FBI)
    b. Food and Drug Administration (FDA)
    c. Department of Health and Human Services (HHS)
    d. Drug Enforcement Administration (DEA)
    e. United States Pharmacopeia (USP)

4. A pharmacist wants to know if generic warfarin tablets are bioequivalent to brand name Coumadin tablets. Where can this information be found?
   a. The Purple Book
   b. The Blue Book
   c. The Green Book
   d. The Orange Book
   e. The Red Book

5. When a pharmacy submits a DEA Form 222 (single sheet) to purchase Schedule II controlled substances, who keeps the original copy of the DEA Form 222?
   a. The pharmacy
   b. The supplier
   c. The manufacturer
   d. The DEA
   e. The pharmacist

6. Which DEA form must be completed and submitted to the DEA upon discovering a theft or significant loss of controlled substances?
   a. DEA Form 106
   b. DEA Form 108
   c. DEA Form 222
   d. DEA Form 224
   e. DEA Form 363

7. What is the first application that must be submitted to the FDA before a drug can be administered to humans in order to start testing?
   a. Supplemental New Drug Application (SNDA)
   b. Investigational New Drug Application (IND)
   c. New Drug Application (NDA)
   d. Abbreviated New Drug Application (ANDA)
   e. Experimental New Drug Application (ENDA)

8. Which phase of a clinical trial is first used to determine the efficacy of a drug?
   a. Phase I
   b. Phase II
   c. Phase III
   d. Phase IV
   e. Phase V

9. What Act regulates the sale and recordkeeping requirements for prescription drug samples?
   a. Prescription Drug Marketing Act
   b. Durham-Humphrey Amendment
   c. Pure Food and Drug Act
   d. Food, Drug and Cosmetic Act
   e. Kefauver-Harris Amendment

10. A manufacturer has a drug that is currently on the market, but they want to change the way the drug is produced. What type of application must be submitted to the FDA in order to request approval for this change?
    a. Prior Approval Supplement (PAS)
    b. Investigational New Drug Application (IND)
    c. New Drug Application (NDA)
    d. Abbreviated New Drug Application (ANDA)
    e. Manufacturer New Drug Application (MNDA)

11. Which FDA expedited review program is intended for drugs that treat serious conditions and fill an unmet medical need?
    a. Breakthrough therapy
    b. Instant approval
    c. Fast track
    d. Accelerated approval
    e. Priority review

12. Schedule II controlled substances CANNOT be transferred in which of the following scenarios?
    a. A pharmacy is closing and decides to transfer their Schedule II controlled substance inventory to another pharmacy
    b. A pharmacy is not renewing their DEA registration and therefore wants to transfer their remaining Schedule II controlled substances to another pharmacy
    c. A pharmacy ordered the wrong Schedule II controlled substances and wants to transfer them back to the supplier
    d. A researcher would like to transfer excess Schedule II controlled substances to a pharmacy to be dispensed to patients
    e. A pharmacy wants to transfer 2 bottles of Schedule II controlled substances to another pharmacy

13. A patient wants to refill a prescription but was not satisfied with the pharmacy that filled and dispensed the prescription the first time. The patient demands the prescription be returned so they can take it to a different pharmacy to obtain refills. The pharmacist should:
    a. Document the original fill information on the original prescription, keep a copy, and return the original prescription to the patient
    b. Offer to give a copy of the prescription to the patient, keep the original copy at the pharmacy, and recommend the patient request the prescription be transferred to another pharmacy if legal
    c. Void the original prescription before returning it to the patient and offer to transfer the rest verbally to another pharmacy
    d. Document the situation in the patient's profile and return the original prescription to the patient
    e. Inform the patient you can send the prescription by priority mail to the pharmacy of their choice

14. An example of an adulterated drug is:
    a. The name of the manufacturer is not included on the label
    b. A medication that has an unapproved color additive
    c. Active ingredients are missing from the bottle
    d. The drug causes an allergic reaction in the patient
    e. The drug container does not contain proper directions for nonprescription drugs

15. What was the first law requiring drugs to be proven safe before being marketed?
    a. Food, Drug, and Cosmetic Act
    b. Kefauver-Harris Amendment
    c. Pure Food and Drug Act
    d. Prescription Drug Marketing Act
    e. Durham-Humphrey Amendment

16. What set of regulations specifies the required minimum manufacturing standards for pharmaceutical products in the U.S.?
    a. Standards of Manufacturing Practice (SMP)
    b. Good Pharmaceutical Manufacturing Practice (GPMP)
    c. Requirements of Good Manufacturing Practice (RGMP)
    d. Regulations of Manufacturing Practice (RMP)
    e. Good Manufacturing Practice (GMP)

17. A drug has an NDC of 16103-0350-11. The 0350 represents:
    a. The manufacturer name
    b. The amount packaged
    c. The identity of the drug
    d. The location of manufacturing
    e. The type of route of administration

18. Which of the following is a Schedule II controlled substance?
    a. Buprenorphine
    b. Butabarbital
    c. Mescaline
    d. Pentobarbital
    e. Modafinil

19. A prescription for lorazepam can be refilled a maximum of how many times within a six-month period?
    a. Zero
    b. Two
    c. Three
    d. Five
    e. Six

20. Which of the following is NOT required on the manufacturer's drug container label for an oral drug product?
    a. Name of the manufacturer
    b. The expiration date
    c. Name of the drug or product
    d. Directions for administration
    e. The net quantity packaged

21. A water-containing oral formulation that is compounded from commercially available drug products has a maximum beyond-use date (BUD) of _____ when refrigerated.
    a. 3 days
    b. 7 days
    c. 14 days
    d. 30 days
    e. 45 days

22. Which of the following is a mid-level practitioner?
    a. Physician
    b. Dentist
    c. Veterinarian
    d. Optometrist
    e. Podiatrist

23. Durable Medical Equipment (DME) must meet which standards? Select ALL that apply.
    a. It can withstand repeated use
    b. Strictly for assistance with walking
    c. Limited to use for paraplegics
    d. Appropriate for use in the home
    e. It is primarily for a medical purpose

24. Federal investigations into thefts and robberies may take place per the Controlled Substances Registrant Protection Act (CSRPA) if the incident meets which of the following conditions?

    I. It will cost $500 or more to replace controlled substances

    II. An employee suffers from significant injuries or death

    III. Theft occurred during drug transport to the pharmacy

    a. I only
    b. II only
    c. I and II
    d. I and III
    e. I, II, and III

25. What Act set the requirement that patients must be offered counseling on dispensed medications?
    a. OSHA 90
    b. DATA 90
    c. HCFA 90
    d. OPDP 90
    e. OBRA 90

26. Under the iPLEDGE Risk Evaluation and Mitigation Strategy (REMS) for isotretinoin, what is the maximum number of refills that may be authorized on a prescription?
    a. 0 refills
    b. 1 refill
    c. 2 refills
    d. 5 refills
    e. 11 refills

27. In which situation would it be illegal for a pharmacy to compound drugs?
    a. The quantity prepared is reasonable for filling existing and anticipated prescriptions
    b. Dosage forms are sold only to other pharmacies and not physician offices
    c. Ingredients in the compounded drugs meet national standards
    d. The compounded drug is not commercially available
    e. Interstate distribution of compounded drugs is no more than 5% of total prescriptions sold by the pharmacy per year

28. What DEA form is necessary to purchase or transfer Schedule II controlled substances?
    a. DEA Form 108
    b. DEA Form 222
    c. DEA Form 224
    d. DEA Form 225
    e. DEA Form 363

29. While working at a retail pharmacy, a patient calls and says they just got home from the hospital after having broken their leg. The patient cannot make it to the pharmacy to pick up their prescription for a Schedule II controlled substance that is ready to pick up. The patient asks if the pharmacy can mail the prescription to the house (mail delivery). How should the pharmacist respond?
    a. Controlled substance medications cannot be mailed
    b. Only Schedule III–V controlled substances can be mailed
    c. Controlled substances can only be mailed to the prescriber's office for office pickup
    d. The prescription can be sent to the patient through mail
    e. The prescription can be sent to the patient as long as the drug name is listed on the package

30. Which of the following statements is/are true about narrow therapeutic index (NTI) drugs?

    I.   Small differences in the dose or blood concentration may lead to adverse reactions

    II. They are not permitted to be prescribed

    III. They require careful titration or patient monitoring for safe and effective use

    a. I only
    b. II only
    c. I and III only
    d. II and III only
    e. I, II, and III

31. What Act set the requirement for child-resistant closures for prescription drugs, non-prescription drugs, and hazard household products?
    a. Poison Prevention Packaging Act
    b. Child Drug Safety Act
    c. Prevention of Hazardous Consumption Act
    d. Children Poison Prevention Act
    e. Hazardous Materials Safety Act

32. For which type of drug recall is there a possibility of temporary or medically reversible adverse effects, but the probability of serious adverse effects is remote?
    a. Class I
    b. Class II
    c. Class III
    d. Class A
    e. Class B

33. What types of patients are included in a Phase I clinical trial for drug development?
    a. Large group of non-human animals
    b. Small group of healthy participants without the disease condition
    c. Small group of participants with the disease condition
    d. Large group of healthy participants without the disease condition
    e. Large group of participants with the disease condition

34. Re-importation of medications is only legal if performed by the:

    I. Retail pharmacy

    II. Original manufacturer

    III. Wholesale distributor

    a. I only
    b. II only
    c. III only
    d. I and III only
    e. I, II, and III

35. What law requires drugs to be proven effective (as well as safe) before being marketed?
    a. Durham-Humphrey Amendment
    b. Pure Food and Drug Act
    c. Prescription Drug Marketing Act
    d. Hatch-Waxman Amendment
    e. Kefauver-Harris Amendment

36. Which DEA registration form is used for pharmacies to register with the DEA to possess and dispense controlled substances?
    a. DEA Form 108
    b. DEA Form 222
    c. DEA Form 224
    d. DEA Form 225
    e. DEA Form 363

37. What information is required to be included in the transaction report transmitted from a manufacturer to a pharmacy when the pharmacy purchases bulk bottles of a medication?
    a. Transaction information, Transaction history, Transaction log
    b. Transaction purpose, Transaction history, Transaction ID number
    c. Transaction information, Transaction history, Transaction statement
    d. Transaction ID number, Transaction code, Transaction statement
    e. Transaction purpose, Transaction history, Transaction log

38. A pharmacist receives an urgent notification from a manufacturing company for a recall of a specific medication because it may cause serious adverse health issues or death. What type of drug recall is this?
    a. Class I
    b. Class II
    c. Class III
    d. Class IV
    e. Class V

39. What Act requires health care facilities to report death or injuries caused by or suspected to have been caused by a medical device to the FDA or the manufacturer?
    a. FDA Modernization Act
    b. Medical Device Inspection Act
    c. Safe Medical Device Act
    d. Pure Food and Drug Act
    e. The Omnibus Budget Reconciliation Act

40. An example of a misbranded manufacturer's container of a drug would be:
    a. The drug causes an allergic reaction in the patient
    b. The container is made of a substance that leaches into the medication
    c. There is no quantity of the contents listed on the container
    d. The drug is exposed to unsanitary conditions
    e. The patient writes the indication for the medication on their prescription bottle

41. Which of the following is true regarding the stocking and dispensing of methadone at retail pharmacies?
    a. Methadone may not be stocked or dispensed from a retail pharmacy; patients must obtain methadone from a narcotic treatment facility
    b. Methadone may be stocked at a retail pharmacy, but may only be dispensed as an analgesic
    c. Methadone may be stocked at a retail pharmacy, but may only be dispensed for narcotic dependence
    d. Methadone may be stocked at a retail pharmacy, and may be dispensed as either an analgesic or for the short-term treatment of narcotic dependence
    e. Methadone may be stocked at any pharmacy, and may be dispensed as either an analgesic or for the long-term treatment of narcotic dependence

42. According to the FDA, a drug is considered to be an orphan drug if it is for rare diseases or conditions that impact fewer than how many people in the U.S.?
    a. 10
    b. 500
    c. 200,000
    d. 1,000,000
    e. 2,000,000

43. Which of the following ingredients has special labeling requirements if it is included in a product?
    a. Gelatin
    b. FD&C Yellow No. 5
    c. High fructose corn syrup
    d. Sorbitol
    e. Xanthan gum

44. In which case(s) is it appropriate to receive a faxed prescription for a Schedule II controlled substance?

    I.   Patient is a resident of a long-term care facility (LTCF)

    II. Patient is enrolled in hospice program

    III. Medication is intended for home infusion therapy

    a. I only
    b. II only
    c. I and II
    d. II and III
    e. I, II, and III

45. What is the acronym of the voluntary reporting system for medication adverse events?
    a. VAERS
    b. FAERS
    c. ERSA
    d. MAERS
    e. AERS

46. Within how many days must a prescriber deliver a written prescription for a Schedule II controlled substance that was called in orally to be dispensed in an emergency situation?
    a. 3 days
    b. 5 days
    c. 7 days
    d. 14 days
    e. 15 days

47. A pharmacy intern wants to know where to find information on therapeutic equivalence between biologics. Which book contains this information?
    a. Red Book
    b. Purple Book
    c. Pink Book
    d. Orange Book
    e. Yellow Book

48. In which case(s) must an exact count be taken while performing a controlled substance inventory?

    I. It is a Schedule II controlled substance

    II. The bottle holds more than 1000 tablets or capsules

    III. Containers are sealed or unopened

    a. I only
    b. II only
    c. I and II
    d. II and III
    e. I, II, and III

49. The scheduling of controlled substances at the federal level is performed by the:
    a. Food and Drug Administration
    b. U.S. Attorney General
    c. Drug Enforcement Agency
    d. National Board of Pharmacy
    e. Drug Enforcement Administration

50. A manufacturer of a prescription-only drug wants to reclassify the drug as an over-the-counter (OTC) drug. What is one of the forms that may be submitted to the FDA when requesting reclassification of a prescription-only drug to an over-the-counter drug?
    a. Emergency Investigational New Drug Application (EIND)
    b. Investigational New Drug Application (IND)
    c. New Drug Application (NDA)
    d. Abbreviated New Drug Application (ANDA)
    e. Marketed New Drug Application (MNDA)

51. You are a pharmacist that suspects a fake controlled substance prescription was called in to your pharmacy. You use the numbers in the provided DEA to verify if it is a true DEA number. It is indeed not a true DEA number because the last number is incorrect. The DEA number is BS5927683. What would be the correct last digit of the DEA number if it was accurate?
    a. 1
    b. 2
    c. 4
    d. 5
    e. 6

52. Which of the following prescriptions would likely be out of the scope of practice for a dentist?
    a. Tylenol #3
    b. Amoxicillin
    c. Lorazepam
    d. Atorvastatin
    e. None of the above; dentists are not limited to scope of practice

53. Who is authorized to sign a DEA 222 Form at a community pharmacy?
    a. Any pharmacist
    b. Any pharmacist or technician
    c. Only the pharmacist-in-charge
    d. Only the pharmacist who signed the most recent application for renewal of the pharmacy's DEA registration
    e. The pharmacist who signed the most recent application for renewal of the pharmacy's DEA registration or someone authorized under a power of attorney

54. Over-the-counter (OTC) drug advertising is regulated by the:
    a. Federal Trade Commission
    b. Food and Drug Administration
    c. Drug Quality and Security Commission
    d. Consumer Product Safety Commission
    e. None of the above

55. A pharmacy may keep which of the following records at a central location other than the location registered with the DEA?
    a. Controlled substance inventories
    b. Controlled substance prescriptions
    c. Controlled substance shipping and financial records
    d. Copies of executed DEA form 222 orders
    e. None of the above may be kept at a central location, all must be kept at the pharmacy

56. Acetaminophen with codeine (Tylenol #3) is classified under which controlled substance schedule?
    a. Schedule I
    b. Schedule II
    c. Schedule III
    d. Schedule IV
    e. Schedule V

57. A patient is admitted to a hospital and does not remember the names of the medications that she takes at home. The hospital pharmacist calls the patient's outpatient pharmacy to obtain a list of medications. Which of the following statements is true?
    a. This is a HIPAA violation unless the patient has given signed consent for the information to be given to the hospital
    b. This is a HIPAA violation unless the patient has given verbal consent for the information to be given to the hospital
    c. This is a HIPAA violation unless the patient has given written and verbal consent for the information to be given to the hospital
    d. This is not a HIPAA violation because HIPAA does not apply to patients being treated in a hospital setting
    e. This is not a HIPAA violation because the information is being given to the hospital for treatment purposes

58. A warning stating "Caution: Federal law prohibits the transfer of this drug to any person other than the patient for whom it was prescribed" is required on the label on which of the following prescriptions?
    a. Schedule II controlled substances only
    b. Schedule II–IV controlled substances only
    c. Schedule II–V controlled substances only
    d. Schedule III–V controlled substances only
    e. All prescriptions require this warning under federal law

59. Registering with the FDA as an outsourcing facility allows a pharmacy to:
    a. Compound sterile products without receiving patient-specific prescriptions
    b. Act as a mail order pharmacy with the ability to send medications to multiple states
    c. Process prescriptions and medication orders remotely for another pharmacy, but not dispense any medications
    d. Repackage medications so that they can be used at hospitals and other institutions
    e. Order drug products listed on the FDA drug shortage list at a discounted cost

60. According to federal law, how may a pharmacy file paper prescription records? Select ALL that apply.
    a. 3 buckets: Schedule II, Schedule III–V, non-controlled
    b. 2 buckets: Schedule II–V (red "C" on Schedule III–V), non-controlled
    c. 1 bucket: All prescriptions filed together regardless of their controlled status
    d. 2 buckets: Schedule II, Schedule III–V and non-controlled (red "C" on Schedule III–V)
    e. 3 buckets: Schedule II–III, Schedule IV–V, non-controlled

61. Standards and requirements for preparing sterile compounded drugs to ensure patient benefit and reduce risks such as contamination, infection, or incorrect dosing are outlined in which of the following?
    a. USP Chapter <503A>
    b. USP Chapter <503B>
    c. USP Chapter <795>
    d. USP Chapter <797>
    e. USP Chapter <800>

62. Which of the following is/are required to register with the Drug Enforcement Administration (DEA)? Select ALL that apply.
    a. A patient who receives a prescription for a controlled substance
    b. A manufacturer that manufactures controlled substances
    c. A pharmacy that dispenses controlled substances
    d. A physician who prescribes controlled substances
    e. A pharmacist who dispenses controlled substances

63. Which of the following medications requires Risk Evaluation and Mitigation Strategy (REMS) monitoring?
    a. Hydromorphone (Dilaudid)
    b. Clozapine (Clozaril)
    c. Fluoxetine (Prozac)
    d. Zolpidem (Ambien)
    e. Metformin (Glucophage)

64. A DEA Form 41 is used to document which of the following?
    a. Purchasing of controlled substances from a manufacturer
    b. Transfer of controlled substances to a reverse distributor
    c. On-site destruction of controlled substances
    d. Significant loss or theft of controlled substances
    e. None of the above

65. What Act set the requirement for tamper-evident packaging for some over-the-counter products in order to avoid risk of contamination?
    a. Safe Drug Packaging Act
    b. Federal Anti-Tampering Act
    c. Drug Contamination Prevention Act
    d. Federal Anti-Contamination Act
    e. Tamper-Evident Packaging Act

66. Drugs that have a high potential for abuse and severe potential for dependence with no currently accepted medical use in the U.S. are classified as:
    a. Schedule I
    b. Schedule II
    c. Schedule III
    d. Schedule IV
    e. None of the above

67. Which of the following is NOT required to be included on a manufacturer's container of an over-the-counter (OTC) medication?
    a. Warnings
    b. Inactive ingredients
    c. Poison Control Center phone number
    d. Purpose
    e. Directions

68. A nursing home patient who is prescribed an estrogen-containing product must be given a Patient Package Insert (PPI):
    a. Prior to the first administration only
    b. Prior to the first administration and every 30 days thereafter
    c. Prior to the first administration and every 60 days thereafter
    d. Only when requested by the patient
    e. None of the above

69. For how long is a DEA registration for possession of controlled substances valid?
    a. 12 months
    b. 24 months
    c. 36 months
    d. 48 months
    e. 60 months

70. Which of the following statements is/are true regarding DEA Form 222?

    I.   Executed copies of DEA Form 222 must be maintained separately from all other records.

    II. A defective DEA Form 222 may be corrected and reused.

    III. On the DEA Form 222, only 1 item may be entered on each numbered line.

    a. I only
    b. II only
    c. I and III only
    d. II and III only
    e. I, II, and III

71. An independent community pharmacy wants to start offering refill reminders to patients in the form of a postcard mailed to the patient's house. The fee for this service would be $2 per month. Which of the following is true regarding this service?
    a. This service cannot be provided because it creates a HIPAA violation
    b. Signed authorization would be required from each patient, as this is considered use of protected health information (PHI) for marketing purposes
    c. This service does not violate HIPAA, but patients cannot be charged a fee for refill reminders
    d. This service does not violate HIPAA, but the reminders must be transmitted electronically
    e. There are no barriers to offering this service and the pharmacy can proceed as planned

72. The expiration date on a bottle of metformin purchased from a manufacturer by a pharmacy is listed as 03/22. What is the expiration date of the drug?
    a. March 1, 2022
    b. March 19, 2022
    c. March 30, 2022
    d. March 31, 2022
    e. None of the above

73. A prospective drug utilization review (DUR) consists of reviewing all of the following aspects of a prescription EXCEPT for:
    a. Underutilization
    b. Therapeutic duplication
    c. Compliance with prescription labeling
    d. Appropriate dosing and regimen
    e. Drug interactions

74. Which of the following statements is required on an over-the-counter (OTC) package of acetaminophen tablets under the Federal Hazardous Substances Act?
    a. "Keep out of the reach of children"
    b. "Consult a doctor before use"
    c. "Do not use if pregnant or breastfeeding"
    d. "Prescription not required"
    e. "For adult use only"

75. A pharmacy dispenses and distributes a total of 50,000 doses of controlled substances in a 12-month period. How many doses is the pharmacy able to transfer to another pharmacy without registering as a distributor?
    a. 500 doses
    b. 1,000 doses
    c. 2,500 doses
    d. 5,000 doses
    e. 10,000 doses

76. The Occupational and Safety Health Administration (OSHA) requires that pharmacies do which of the following?
    a. Provide patients with information regarding the safe handling of hazardous medications
    b. Provide patients with Safety Data Sheets for hazardous medications
    c. Include the word "caution" or "warning" on labels for all hazardous medications
    d. Train all of their employees on the hazards of chemicals and on the protective measures they should take
    e. None of the above

77. The Poison Prevention Packaging Act (PPPA), which requires child-resistant containers for prescription and certain non-prescription drugs (with some exceptions), is administered by the:
    a. Food and Drug Administration
    b. Consumer Product Safety Commission
    c. Federal Trade Commission
    d. Centers for Medicare and Medicaid Services
    e. Occupational and Safety Health Administration

78. A pharmacy orders bulk bottles of ibuprofen and compounds ibuprofen suppositories. These suppositories are sold to other pharmacies that need to fill prescriptions but do not have the ability to make them. Which of the following terms best describes this practice?
    a. Compounding
    b. Dispensing
    c. Bulk compounding
    d. Manufacturing
    e. Outsourcing

79. Which of the following is true regarding the purchasing and selling of prescription drug samples?
    a. Drug samples may be purchased by a community pharmacy from a drug company and sold to patients at a standard price set by the FDA
    b. Drug samples may be purchased by a community pharmacy but must be given to patients free of charge
    c. Drug samples may only be given to a patient at a community pharmacy if the patient already has a prescription for the same medication
    d. Drug samples may be given to a pharmacy owned by a charitable organization and sold to patients at a reduced cost if the facility provides care to indigent or low-income patients
    e. Drug samples may be given to a pharmacy which is owned by a charitable organization that provides care to indigent or low-income patients, but must be given to patients free of charge

80. Which of the following is a valid method of ordering Schedule III medications from a supplier to restock a pharmacy's bulk medication supply?
    a. Mailing a hard copy of DEA Form 222 to the supplier
    b. Mailing a hard copy of DEA Form 224 to the supplier
    c. Faxing a copy of DEA Form 222 to the supplier
    d. Faxing a copy of DEA Form 224 to the supplier
    e. Sending an online order to the supplier with no additional form sent

81. Which of the following products is NOT required to be in tamper-evident packaging for retail sale?
    a. Acetaminophen tablets
    b. Children's diphenhydramine liquid
    c. Aspirin tablets
    d. Benzocaine/menthol lozenges
    e. Infant simethicone drops

82. A pharmacist may call a prescriber and receive verbal permission to change all of the following on a Schedule II prescription EXCEPT:
    a. Quantity
    b. Directions for use
    c. Drug name
    d. Drug strength
    e. Dosage form

83. A patient requests a copy of her prescription records from a community pharmacy. Within what time period must the pharmacy provide this information?
    a. 24 hours
    b. 3 days
    c. 7 days
    d. 10 days
    e. 30 days

84. Which of the following drugs has a REMS program due to a high frequency of birth defects?
    a. Lisinopril
    b. Thalidomide
    c. Zyprexa
    d. Atorvastatin
    e. Levothyroxine

85. Which law requires new drugs to be proven as safe and effective before approval?
    a. Poison Prevention Packaging Act
    b. Durham-Humphrey Amendment
    c. Kefauver-Harris Amendment
    d. Prescription Drug Marketing Act
    e. Drug Quality and Security Act

86. Anabolic steroids are classified under which controlled substance schedule under federal law?
    a. Schedule I
    b. Schedule II
    c. Schedule III
    d. Schedule IV
    e. Schedule V

87. Which Act or Amendment created the separation of drugs into two different categories, prescription (legend) and over-the-counter?
    a. Kefauver-Harris Amendment
    b. Omnibus Reconciliation Act
    c. Hatch-Waxman Amendment
    d. Durham-Humphrey Amendment
    e. Robinson-Patman Act

88. A patient picks up a prescription for Xarelto at a community pharmacy, but returns later in the day concerned that the prescription was filled with generic rivaroxaban. The pharmacist explains that the prescription was filled with the generic form of the medication because it was cheaper than using the brand name product. The patient asks if the generic will work as well as the brand name product. According to the pharmacist's drug reference, the two products have an FDA equivalency rating of AB. What is the proper interpretation of this code?

    a. The products are not bioequivalent, and the prescription should be filled only with brand name Xarelto
    b. The products have not been studied to determine bioequivalence, so a determination cannot be made
    c. The products have no known or suspected bioequivalence issues and are interchangeable
    d. The products may have actual or potential bioequivalence issues, but there is adequate evidence to use them interchangeably
    e. The code AB alone does not provide enough information to determine bioequivalence

89. DEA registration is NOT required for which of the following situations? Select ALL that apply.

    a. A nurse who is working in a physician's office where controlled substances are prescribed
    b. A pharmacist who regularly dispenses controlled substances at a community pharmacy
    c. A physician who prescribes controlled substances at a private clinic
    d. A patient who picks up a prescription for a newly prescribed controlled substance
    e. A pharmacy dispensing controlled substances

90. A drug manufacturer finds that bottles labeled "loratadine 10mg tablets" actually contain 5mg tablets, and issues a recall of the affected lot. Which of the following is true of this product?

    a. It is adulterated
    b. It is misbranded
    c. It is contaminated
    d. It is both adulterated and misbranded
    e. None of the above

91. A physician writes a prescription for ibuprofen 800mg tablets for a patient with rheumatoid arthritis. On the prescription, the physician adds a note that says, "please place this prescription and all future prescriptions in easy-open containers, as the patient is unable to open child-resistant bottles." Which of the following is true regarding this request?
    a. It is not valid because providers do not have the authority to request special packaging on a patient's behalf
    b. It is not valid because ibuprofen is not on the list of drugs exempt from the child-resistant packaging requirement under the Poison Prevention Packaging Act
    c. It is not valid because the provider must submit a separate signed form to make this request
    d. The ibuprofen can be dispensed in an easy-open container, but the blanket request to provide easy-open caps on all future prescriptions is not valid because only the patient can make such a request
    e. It is valid and a note should be made on the patient's profile to use easy-open containers on all prescriptions in the future

92. Which of the following would NOT be considered a potential part of a Risk Evaluation and Mitigation Strategy (REMS) program?
    a. Requiring special certification for pharmacies, practitioners, or health care settings that dispense a drug
    b. Requiring laboratory testing to ensure safe use of a drug
    c. Performing a financial assessment to ensure that a patient can afford a drug for the duration of treatment
    d. Providing a Medication Guide to patients which includes information about a drug
    e. Requiring that a patient enroll in a registry when they begin taking a drug

93. Retail containers of chewable low-dose 81mg aspirin (1.25 grain) must have special warnings for use in children including a warning regarding Reye's syndrome, and cannot contain more than:
    a. 10 tablets
    b. 30 tablets
    c. 36 tablets
    d. 48 tablets
    e. 60 tablets

94. Which of these is a valid DEA Registration number for a mid-level practitioner?
    a. M11496023
    b. MT1200980
    c. CR5624112
    d. MM7411222
    e. BL115231

95. The FDA may require a Medication Guide (MedGuide) be issued with certain prescriptions for which reasons? Select ALL that apply.
    a. When a drug has serious risks relative to benefits
    b. When patient adherence is crucial
    c. When the patient is a resident of a nursing home or other institution
    d. When drug information can prevent serious adverse effects
    e. When a pharmacist is unavailable to provide counseling on a new prescription

96. Which of the following can be determined from the National Drug Code (NDC) number on a medication bottle? Select ALL that apply.
    a. Manufacturer
    b. Specific drug
    c. Package
    d. Expiration date
    e. FDA approval status

97. Which of the following is/are NOT required to be packaged in a child-resistant container? Select ALL that apply.
    a. A container of 30 sublingual nitroglycerin tablets
    b. A methylprednisolone dose pack containing 21 tablets that are 4mg each
    c. A container of 100 aspirin tablets
    d. A prednisone dose pack containing 21 tablets that are 10mg each
    e. An albuterol inhaler

98. Prescription records must be kept for a minimum of _____ based on federal law.
    a. 1 year
    b. 2 years
    c. 3 years
    d. 4 years
    e. 5 years

99. In the event of a breach of unsecured protected health information (PHI) at a retail pharmacy affecting approximately 900 patients, who must be notified? Select ALL that apply.
    a. All nearby pharmacies
    b. Prominent local media outlets
    c. Affected patients
    d. All patients who use the pharmacy
    e. U.S. Secretary of Health and Human Services (HHS)

100. To comply with Centers for Medicare and Medicaid Services (CMS) requirements, how often must a pharmacist conduct a Drug Regimen Review for long-term care patients?
    a. At least once a week
    b. At least once a month
    c. At least once every 60 days
    d. At least once every 6 months
    e. Annually

Kentucky MPJE Practice Questions

1. A pharmacy in the state of Kentucky is scheduled to receive a shipment of legend drugs that includes controlled substances. The shipment did not arrive on the anticipated date of delivery. The pharmacy should report the nonreceipt of the shipment:
   a. Immediately upon notice of nonreceipt
   b. Within three business days of discussion with shipper, if still not received
   c. Within three business days of anticipated receipt date
   d. Within five business days of discussion with shipper, if still not received
   e. Within five business days of anticipated receipt date

2. Out of state pharmacies are required to:
   a. Provide a toll-free telephone service directly to the pharmacist in charge 24/7
   b. Provide an electronic e-mail service directly to the pharmacist in charge 24/7
   c. Provide a toll-free telephone service directly to the pharmacist in charge during regular hours of operation
   d. Provide an electronic e-mail service directly to the pharmacist in charge during regular hours of operation
   e. Provide both a toll-free telephone service and an electronic email service directly to the pharmacist in charge not less than 6 days per week and for a minimum 40 hours per week

3. Any pharmacy within the state of Kentucky doing business primarily or exclusively by the use of the internet must be certified that it is a:
   a. PMPI
   b. CFR
   c. VIPPS
   d. KYCP
   e. CAMP

4. Which of the following is/are required when someone is applying for a pharmacy license?

   I. Be 18 years of age or older

   II. Graduate from a college of pharmacy approved by the Board

   III. Complete the requirements of internship

   a. I only
   b. II only
   c. I and II only
   d. I and III only
   e. I, II, and III

5. How long must pharmacists keep valid records, receipts, and certifications of completed continuing pharmacy education programs?
   a. 1 year
   b. 2 years
   c. 3 years
   d. 5 years
   e. 6 years

6. How many continuing education units (CEU) are required by each pharmacist every year under Kentucky State Pharmacy law?
   a. 1.5
   b. 3.0
   c. 10
   d. 15
   e. 30

7. How many years are certificates of internship valid?
    a. One year
    b. Two years
    c. Four years
    d. Six years
    e. Eight years

8. In the Commonwealth of Kentucky, on what date does a license to practice pharmacy expire every year?
    a. January 1
    b. February 28
    c. June 30
    d. September 30
    e. December 31

9. What is true regarding renewal of a pharmacist's license in the state of Kentucky?
    a. A pharmacist that fails to comply with renewal requirements will be notified by the executive director within 30 days after the renewal period closes.
    b. A pharmacist who failed to renew their license for any consecutive period up to 5 years may renew their license only after satisfying the continuing education regulations of the Board and paying the cumulative penalty and renewal fees.
    c. A pharmacist who failed to renew their license for 5 consecutive years or more may renew their license only upon satisfying the continuing education regulations of the Board, passing a satisfactory examination before the Board and paying the renewal and penalty fees.
    d. An inactive license holder can apply for an active license and must pay a renewal fee not exceeding fifty dollars.
    e. All of the above

10. A licensee, permit holder or certificate holder who is disciplined for a minor violation of regulations can request in writing that the Board expunge the minor violation from their permanent record after how long?
    a. Six months
    b. One year
    c. Two years
    d. Three years
    e. Four years

11. The Board may suspend a pharmacist license for which of the following reasons?

    I. Failing to notify the Board within 14 days of a change in home address

    II. Failing to repay a student loan

    III. Failing to report that a pharmacist is incapable of engaging in the practice of pharmacy

    a. I only
    b. II only
    c. I and II only
    d. I and III only
    e. I, II, and III

12. The pharmacist recovery network committee is comprised of:
    a. 3 members
    b. 5 members
    c. 7 members
    d. 9 members
    e. 11 members

13. What is the maximum amount of Robitussin A/C that can be dispensed within a 48-hour period?
    a. 240 cc
    b. 120 cc
    c. 60 cc
    d. 480 cc
    e. 180 cc

14. The Board must establish which of the following to promote early identification, intervention, treatment and rehabilitation of pharmacists or pharmacist interns who may be impaired due to reasons of illness, alcohol or drug abuse?
    a. Pharmacist Support Resources Committee
    b. Pharmacist Helping Hand and Rehabilitation Association
    c. Pharmacist Health and Recovery Organization
    d. Pharmacist Recovery Network Committee
    e. Pharmacist Mental Health and Rehabilitation Association

15. The Board may temporarily suspend a license, certificate, or permit, without benefit of a hearing, if the president of the Board finds that the individual:
    a. Has violated a statute or administrative regulation the Board is empowered to enforce
    b. Is dangerous to the health, welfare, and safety of the general public
    c. Has a mental or physical condition that through continued practice could create imminent risk or harm to the public
    d. The Board cannot suspend a license, certificate, or permit without a hearing
    e. a, b, and c

16. A person may assist in the practice of pharmacy without obtaining the technician registration required by the Board if the person: (select ALL that apply)
    a. Has filed an application with the Board and no more than thirty days has elapsed since the date the applicant was first employed by the pharmacy
    b. Is participating in a work-study program through an accredited secondary or postsecondary educational institution
    c. Has filed an application that has been rejected, and is awaiting an appeal decision by the Board
    d. Is employed by a son, daughter, spouse, parent, or legal guardian
    e. Is awaiting approval of transitioning their technician registration to a pharmacist intern license

17. What are requirements to become a registered pharmacy technician under the Kentucky State Pharmacy Law? (select ALL that apply)
    a. Applicants must be 18 years of age and older
    b. Applicants must be of good mental health
    c. Applicants must be of good moral character
    d. Applicants must hold a high school diploma or General Education Diploma equivalent
    e. Applicants must pay a registration fee not more than $25

18. How long can a Kentucky State Board of Pharmacy member serve throughout their lifetime?
    a. Two years
    b. Four years
    c. Six Years
    d. Eight years
    e. Ten years

19. What is true regarding pharmacy technician registration?
    a. The pharmacy technician's certificate of registration must be located within a pharmacy's administrative files
    b. A pharmacy technician must complete 1.5 CEU to obtain a registration renewal
    c. Pharmacy technician registration must be renewed on or before February 28 of each year
    d. A pharmacy technician must pay a $25 registration renewal fee but need not submit a renewal application
    e. Delinquent renewals are subject to a penalty fee for each renewal period the registrant fails to remove their registration after expiration

20. How many pharmacists serve on the Kentucky State Board of Pharmacy?
    a. Two
    b. Three
    c. Four
    d. Five
    e. Six

21. When can a pharmacist substitute a generic equivalent drug for a prescription order?
    a. The brand name is written on the prescription and the pharmacist substitutes a lower cost generic equivalent
    b. The brand name is written on the prescription along with "Do Not Substitute" and the pharmacist substitutes a lower cost generic equivalent
    c. The brand name is written on the prescription and the pharmacist substitutes a higher cost generic equivalent
    d. The brand name for a biological product is written and the pharmacist substitutes a noninterchangeable product
    e. The brand name is written on the prescription and the generic name is in the nonequivalent drug product formulary prepared by the Board

22. How often is the Kentucky State Board of Pharmacy required to meet?
    a. Annually
    b. Twice a year
    c. Four times a year
    d. Every other month
    e. Monthly

23. Who appoints members to serve on the Kentucky State Board of Pharmacy?
    a. The Governor
    b. The Executive Director
    c. The President of the Board
    d. The Mayor from the city of the appointed member
    e. The President of the Cabinet for Health & Family Services

24. The Governor may remove a Board member for which of the following reasons:

    I. Inability of the Board member to perform his duties in an efficient, responsible or professional manner

    II. Violation of any provision of KRS Chapter 315 or any regulation set forth thereunder

    III. Misuse of the office to obtain personal, pecuniary, or material gain for himself or another

    a. I only
    b. I and II
    c. I and III
    d. II and III
    e. I, II, and III

25. Under Kentucky State Pharmacy Law, what organization is an approved continuing education provider?

    I. The Accreditation Council for Pharmacy Education (ACPE)

    II. Kentucky Pharmacy Board

    III. Accredited school of pharmacy continuing education programs

    a. I only
    b. I and II only
    c. II and III only
    d. I and III only
    e. All of the above

26. Which of the following is true regarding the use of automated pharmacy systems in a residential hospice facility? (select ALL that apply)
    a. A licensed pharmacist must supervise the use of the system
    b. The pharmacist can remotely monitor the system by electronic means
    c. An automated pharmacy system may not dispense legend drugs
    d. Drugs must be prepared in unit dose packaging
    e. The Board can declare regulations regarding the accuracy and security of automated systems

27. A charitable pharmacy may:
    a. Dispense controlled substances
    b. Only dispense prescriptions to qualified indigent populations
    c. Accept previously opened or partial use stock bottles of legend drug products
    d. Operate without routine application for a permit, since it does not service all patients
    e. Charge a reduced or discounted fee for prescriptions dispensed

28. According to Kentucky Pharmacy Statutes and Regulations, a pharmacy is allowed to place drugs with a home health agency's authorized employees and with a hospice's authorized employees for the betterment of public health. What legend drug is allowed under this agreement?
    a. Insulin regular injectable
    b. Glucagon
    c. Heparin subcutaneous injectable
    d. Ketorolac injectable
    e. Tetanus, diphtheria, pertussis vaccine

29. What is FALSE regarding continuing education requirements in the state of Kentucky?
    a. A pharmacist must complete a minimum of 1.5 contact hours annually
    b. A pharmacist licensed by the Board within 12 months preceding the renewal date is exempt from CE for that year
    c. A pharmacist can obtain deferral for CE based on the discretion of the Board for illness or incapacity
    d. CE can be transferred from out of state if the transfer state recognizes Kentucky CEU
    e. A pharmacist is required to inform the Board of their correct address

30. What information must be provided when reporting the theft, robbery or loss of a controlled substance? (select ALL that apply)
    a. Name, NDC, and quantity of controlled substances involved
    b. Name of pharmacist who identified the discrepancy
    c. Description of circumstances of the loss
    d. Name and description of suspected persons committing the offense or causing the loss
    e. DEA form 106

31. What is true regarding the return or exchange of a legend drug? (select ALL that apply)
    a. Prescription drug products cannot be re-sold after return or exchange
    b. A drug product can only be returned to the original manufacturer
    c. Any person, pharmacy, or pharmacy warehouse authorized to distribute prescription drugs can initiate a drug return or exchange
    d. Manufacturers and wholesalers must only supply prescription drugs to entities licensed for drug distribution
    e. Pharmacies, distributors or those authorized to distribute prescription drugs are held accountable to not permit the acceptance of adulterated or counterfeit drugs by the manufacturer

32. What does an expungement mean according to the Kentucky Administrative Regulation?
    a. Affected records must be sealed
    b. The proceedings the records refer to are deemed to not have occurred once expunged
    c. The affected party will have no records regarding the matter expunged
    d. The affected party will not be the subject of a subsequent violation of the same nature for a period of 3 years after completion of disciplinary sanctions for the violation expunged
    e. All of the above

33. A pharmacist-in-charge (PIC) shall (select ALL that apply):
    a. Serve only one pharmacy at a time, unless with explicit written approval
    b. Be present a minimum 15 hours per week to provide supervision
    c. Ensure all pharmacists and interns are currently licensed
    d. File reports of theft or loss to the DEA or Kentucky State Police
    e. Notify the Board within 30 calendar days of changes to the staff or PIC

34. Which of the following is true regarding the need for permits for operation of a pharmacy?
    a. A permit is required for operation of a pharmacy, regardless of the type or physical means of the pharmacy
    b. Pharmacies operated via the Internet do not require a permit
    c. Each pharmacy must submit a permit fee of $1,000
    d. The Board must act upon an application for a permit within 60 days from its submission
    e. Pharmacies operating under the same roof do not need separate permits

35. Which of the following statement(s) is/are true regarding pharmacist interns? (Select ALL that apply.)
    a. An intern must complete 1500 internship hours prior to being licensed as a pharmacist
    b. An application for registration as a pharmacist intern must be filed with the Board
    c. An intern must carry their pharmacist intern identification at all times while on duty
    d. An intern must be actively enrolled in a college or school of pharmacy approved by the Board
    e. Interns must work under a preceptor, who may supervise up to two pharmacist interns at a time

36. Which of the following may a certified pharmacy technician complete under general supervision of a pharmacist?

    I. Initiate or receive telephonic communication concerning refill authorization

    II. Certify for delivery unit dose mobile transport refilled by other technicians

    III. Initiate or receive telephonic communication for a new drug order (verbal order)

    a. I only
    b. II only
    c. I and II only
    d. I and III only
    e. I, II, and III

37. The pharmacist-in-charge of a hospital pharmacy utilizing an automated pharmacy system is responsible for all of the following, EXCEPT:
    a. Ensuring system accuracy prior to dispensing medications for administration to patients
    b. Reviewing medications prior to loading into the automated pharmacy system
    c. Overseeing a quality assurance program to monitor system performance
    d. Communicating to the Board the installation and removal of an automated pharmacy system
    e. Interacting with hospital IT, who oversees the hardware and software security systems

38. What documentation relating to an automated pharmacy dispensing system must be maintained within a hospital pharmacy?

    I.   A description of how the system is used

    II.   Quality assurance procedures used to maintain appropriate use of the system

    III. Policies and procedures for system operation, safety, and security

    IV.   Manufacturer name, model, serial number, software version

    a. I, IV
    b. I, III, IV
    c. II and IV
    d. II, III, and IV
    e. All of the above

39. What is true regarding the transfer of prescription information for any non-controlled substance prescription for the purpose of refill dispensing?
    a. A transfer can be communicated between a pharmacist intern and a certified pharmacy technician
    b. A transfer cannot be communicated to a pharmacist in another state
    c. A transfer can be communicated between a certified pharmacy technician and a licensed pharmacist
    d. A transfer can be communicated between two pharmacist interns
    e. None of the above

40. In Kentucky, a pharmacy providing pharmaceutical compounding services must maintain a patient profile for at least:
    a. 1 year
    b. 2 years
    c. 3 years
    d. 4 years
    e. 5 years

41. What information must be included on the label for a compounded prescription product? (Select ALL that apply)
    a. Patient's full name and address
    b. Name and address of pharmacy
    c. Name, strength, and amount of each active ingredient or drug product
    d. Lot number of each active ingredient or drug product
    e. Beyond use date
    f. Storage requirements

42. What is true regarding the pharmacist recovery network committee?
    a. The committee was created to promote the early identification, intervention and treatment of pharmacists or interns who may be impaired
    b. The committee can utilize reports of impairment for the basis of disciplinary action
    c. The committee is made up of 9 civilian members plus the president and executive director of the Board
    d. The records and proceedings of the committee pertaining to an impaired pharmacist or intern are considered public records and can be subject to court subpoena
    e. The information disclosed by the committee does not need to be authorized by the impaired pharmacist or intern

43. You have substituted generic Prasugrel (Manufacturer: Aurobindo) for the prescribed brand name Effient (Manufacturer: Lilly). What is the appropriate text to place on the dispensing label?
    a. Prasugrel, (Aurobindo)
    b. Prasugrel, Effient (Aurobindo)
    c. Prasugrel Aurobindo, dispensed for Effient
    d. Effient (Lilly), Prasugrel
    e. Effient (Lilly), substituted by Prasugrel

44. What is FALSE regarding pharmacy services in hospitals or other healthcare facilities?
    a. The pharmacy must be directed by a licensed pharmacist
    b. Labeling and packaging of medications used for outpatients must comply with state laws since federal labeling laws aren't applicable in these facilities
    c. The pharmacy must maintain current drug information and toxicology reference materials
    d. Whenever possible, medications should be dispensed by unit dose distribution
    e. Floor stock of drug product should remain as small as possible

45. What information should be recorded by the pharmacist transferring a prescription in the Commonwealth of Kentucky? (select ALL that apply)
    a. Date of transfer
    b. Name and address of the pharmacy to which it was transferred
    c. Phone number of the pharmacy to which is was transferred
    d. That the prescription is void
    e. Name of pharmacist receiving the prescription information

46. What information should be recorded by the pharmacist receiving a transferred prescription in the Commonwealth of Kentucky? (select ALL that apply)
    a. Date of transfer
    b. Date of issuance of original prescription
    c. Date of original dispensing
    d. Date of last refill
    e. Date of next available refill

47. A newly hired pharmacy technician is processing return-to-stock prescriptions that have been filled but not picked up. They return a prescription vial of atorvastatin tablets to a large stock bottle. The returned tablets are of different lot number and expiration date. Unknowingly, the pharmacist uses this stock bottle of mixed medication to dispense an atorvastatin prescription to a new patient. The newly filled atorvastatin prescription is considered:
    a. Misbranded
    b. Adulterated
    c. Repackaged
    d. Mislabeled
    e. Contaminated

48. An emergency oral prescription for Schedule II controlled drugs must be mailed to dispensing pharmacy by an authorized prescriber within:
    a. 24 hours after an oral authorization
    b. 48 hours after an oral authorization
    c. 72 hours after an oral authorization
    d. 7 days after an oral authorization
    e. 10 days after an oral authorization

49. What is true about refilling a prescription when the prescription has no refills remaining and refill authorization is unable to be obtained from the prescriber?

    I.   The pharmacist can fill the prescription if the drug (or device) is required for continuation of therapy for chronic conditions

    II. The pharmacist can fill the prescription if they determine interruption of therapy may produce serious adverse health consequences

    III. The pharmacist can fill the prescription regardless of control status if the drug (or device) is life sustaining

    IV. The pharmacist obtains an authorization from the prescriber for continued therapy

    a. I and II
    b. I and III
    c. I, II and III
    d. II, III, and IV
    e. I, II, and IV

50. A physician should discontinue the use of Schedule III or IV amphetamine-like controlled substances for weight loss program if: (select ALL that apply)
    a. The patient does not demonstrate weight loss
    b. The patient doesn't attempt to comply with exercise and/or dietary changes
    c. The body mass index of the patient without a co-morbid condition is < 27 or < 25 with a co-morbid condition
    d. The patient has obtained a controlled substance anorexiant from another provider without the prescriber's knowledge
    e. The patient has regained the weight lost

51. When must a pharmacist offer patient counseling?

    I. Upon presentation of an original prescription order

    II. Upon refill of a prescription, if the pharmacist deems counseling necessary

    III. Once yearly on maintenance prescriptions

    a. I only
    b. II only
    c. I and II only
    d. I and III only
    e. I, II, and III

52. Which of the following duties is the Kentucky State Board of Pharmacy authorized to do?

    I. Employ an executive director, which must be a citizen at large

    II. Set time and place for examinations

    III. Schedule and conduct hearings

    IV. Issue and renew licenses

    a. I only
    b. I and II only
    c. II, III, and IV
    d. III and IV only
    e. All of the above

53. What information does NOT need to be included when counseling a patient on their medication?
    a. The name and description of the drug
    b. Techniques for self-monitoring of therapy
    c. Proper storage
    d. Clinical trial efficacy data
    e. Common and clinically significant adverse effects

54. What information about a Patient Medication Record is NOT true?
    a. A patient record should be maintained for at least 180 days from the date of the last entry
    b. A patient record should include a list of all prescriptions obtained by the patient at that pharmacy location for the past 6 months
    c. A patient record should enable the pharmacist to determine the impact of previously dispensed drugs and known disease conditions upon receiving a new prescription order
    d. A patient record should include individual medical history, if significant
    e. All of the statements above are true

55. The purpose of a prospective drug use review is to: (Select ALL that apply)
    a. Anticipate what new medications a patient may be prescribed
    b. Scan the patient profile for untreated medical conditions
    c. Ensure proper utilization of a newly prescribed medication
    d. Scan the patient profile for drug interactions
    e. Assess a new prescription order

56. According to the Kentucky Administrative Regulations, what is true regarding nuclear pharmacies? Select ALL that apply.
    a. Each nuclear pharmacy must be equipped with at least a microscope, dose calibrator, and a drawing station
    b. Nuclear pharmacies must follow general space requirements for all pharmacies
    c. Nuclear pharmacies should maintain records in accordance with the Radiation Control Branch of the Cabinet for Human Resources
    d. A nuclear pharmacy cannot receive an oral prescription for a radiopharmaceutical
    e. A radiopharmaceutical product should be bare a standard radiation symbol on its outermost container

57. A pharmacist may enter into a collaborative care agreement with a practitioner provided all of the following apply, EXCEPT:
    a. The agreement is in writing
    b. Pharmacists are prohibited from initiating therapy under the agreement
    c. The agreement is signed and dated by all participating parties
    d. Methods for termination are documented in the agreement
    e. Documents are maintained for 5 years after termination of the agreement

58. When operating a nuclear pharmacy, what references are required to be maintained on the premises?

   I.   United States Pharmacopeia–National Formulary with supplements

   II. State statutes and administrative regulations relating to pharmacy

   III. Materials related to the practice of nuclear pharmacy and radiation safety

   IV. Clinical Pharmacology

   a. I and II only
   b. I and III only
   c. II, III, and IV only
   d. III and IV only
   e. I, II, and III only

59. What is true regarding a central filling pharmacy in Kentucky?

   I.   The central refill pharmacy prepares the label for the refill prescription, which clearly identifies the name and address of the pharmacy preparing the product for refill dispensing

   II. The central refill pharmacy must provide the originating pharmacy with written information describing how a patient can contact the central refill pharmacy if the patient has questions about the preparation of the refill

   III. The central refill pharmacy is responsible for ensuring the prescription order has been properly verified by a pharmacist

   IV. The central refill pharmacy needs a written contract with the pharmacy that has custody of the original prescription authorization for refill dispensing

   a. I only
   b. I and II only
   c. II and III only
   d. I, II, and III only
   e. I, II, III and IV

60. A patient comes to your pharmacy and requests a transfer of a prescription for Lyrica from another pharmacy. His patient profile shows that three eligible refills (five refills on original prescription) are left on the prescription. If both pharmacies, transferring and receiving, electronically sharing a real-time online database, how many times can the prescription be transferred?
    a. Once
    b. Maximum three times
    c. As many times as needed until prescription expires
    d. Maximum five times
    e. Cannot be transferred

61. A legend drug repository program may be established by the Kentucky State Board of Pharmacy. Legend drugs may qualify for donation to the repository if they meet all of the following criteria, EXCEPT:
    a. The legend drug is in its original, unopened, sealed, and tamper evident packaging
    b. The legend drug is not classified as a controlled substance
    c. The legend drug is not adulterated, misbranded, or counterfeited
    d. The legend drug is prescribed by a physician, APRN or PA and dispensed by a pharmacist
    e. The legend drug can be resold for profit of the repository program

62. A pharmacist receives a new prescription for ProAir HFA inhaler for a new patient at their pharmacy. The prescriber has indicated "formulary compliance approval" on the prescription. After trying to bill the patient's third party insurance plan, the insurance rejected the claim, indicating that the preferred formulary equivalent is Ventolin HFA. According to Kentucky Administrative Regulations (KAR), the pharmacist should:
    a. Fill the prescription for Ventolin HFA and notify the prescribing physician within 24 hours
    b. Fill the prescription for ProAir and have the patient pay the cash price out of pocket
    c. Call the prescribing physician to obtain approval of filling of a formulary equivalent
    d. Not fill the prescription and have the patient obtain a new prescription for the preferred formulary equivalent
    e. Not fill the prescription because formulary compliance dispensing is prohibited under KAR

63. In order for a pharmacist to be authorized to dispense Naloxone, a physician-approved protocol providing authorization must contain: (select ALL that apply)
    a. Criteria for persons eligible to receive Naloxone
    b. Name, dose, and route of administration of Naloxone product dispensed
    c. Name of pharmacist authorized to dispense
    d. Education provided to the persons receiving Naloxone
    e. Outcome and follow up of persons receiving Naloxone administration

64. Which of the following is NOT required as a part of verbal counseling to persons dispensed a Naloxone prescription by a pharmacist?
    a. Signs of opioid overdose
    b. Strategies to prevent an overdose
    c. Risk factors for opioid overdose
    d. How to administer Naloxone
    e. Required elements of the Naloxone dispensing protocol

65. Who is considered a practitioner under Kentucky Revised Statutes, who are legally authorized to prescribe and administer drugs and devices? (Select ALL that apply)
    a. Medical or osteopathic physicians
    b. Dentists
    c. Advanced practice registered nurses
    d. Veterinarians
    e. Optometrists

66. Every person engaged in the sale of hypodermic syringes or needles in a retail setting must maintain a bound record book that is retained for:
    a. 1 year
    b. 2 years
    c. 3 years
    d. 4 years
    e. 5 years

67. Inventory of controlled substances should be done every:
    a. Year
    b. Two years
    c. Three years
    d. Five years
    e. Seven years

68. What is true of the Drug Addiction Treatment Act? (Select ALL that apply)
    a. It allows qualified physicians to treat opioid addiction at their practice site
    b. It requires qualified physicians to obtain a separate DEA (X-)
    c. Physicians are limited to 50 patients under this act
    d. It restricts prescribing to only methadone and Suboxone
    e. Prescriptions written under the act must be labeled with both DEA numbers of the qualified physician

69. Which of the following is NOT a material required to be maintained at a pharmacy for the purposes of suitable pharmacy practice?
    a. A complete set of metric or apothecary weights
    b. A State and Federal Laws and Regulations reference
    c. An air conditioner
    d. A reference that describes drug interactions
    e. Filtration funnel with filter papers

70. A patient arrives to your pharmacy asking for a refill of his ticagrelor for a recent myocardial infarction. Upon profile review, you find the prescription is out of refills, and the prescriber's office will not reopen for another 48 hours to obtain authorization for continuation of therapy. You tell the patient:
    a. You can fill a 24-hour supply, however the patient will need to await prescriber authorization on the next business day for further quantities
    b. You can fill a 48-hour supply and contact the prescriber Monday to obtain refill authorization
    c. You can fill a 72-hour supply and contact the prescriber Monday to obtain refill authorization
    d. You can fill a 7-day supply and contact the prescriber Monday to obtain refill authorization
    e. You cannot fill a short-term supply without authorization from the prescriber

71. What quantity of schedule II medications can an advanced practice registered nurse (APRN) write a prescription for in the State of Kentucky?
    a. 24-hour supply
    b. 72-hour supply
    c. 7-day supply
    d. 14-day supply
    e. 30-day supply

72. Which of the following is NOT included in the criteria to designate a drug a controlled substance according to the Kentucky Controlled Substances Act?
    a. Relative potential for abuse
    b. Risk to public health
    c. History of abuse
    d. Current pattern of abuse
    e. Cost of parent compound of agent

73. Within how many days can a partially filled prescription for morphine sulfate for a terminally ill patient be completed from the time of initial filling?
    a. 72 hours
    b. 7 days
    c. 14 days
    d. 28 days
    e. 60 days

74. What CANNOT be changed on a schedule II controlled substance prescription?

    I. The patient's name

    II. The drug name

    III. The signature of the practitioner

    IV. The prescribing office's name

    a. I only
    b. I and II only
    c. I, II, and III
    d. II, III, and IV
    e. All of the above

75. How long is a non-controlled substance prescription valid for dispensing?
    a. 180 days from the date of issuance
    b. 90 days from the date of issuance
    c. 365 days from the date of issuance
    d. 30 days from the date of issuance
    e. None of the above

76. Which of the following matches the entity authorized to administer controlled substances with the correct duration of time the entity should maintain records of substances administered?
    a. Physicians: 3 years
    b. Manufacturers: 3 years
    c. Wholesalers: 2 years
    d. Pharmacists: 2 years
    e. Dentists: 3 years

77. You receive an electronic prescription for Tylenol No. 3 for dental pain for patient A on March 1st with 5 refills. After taking the medication for a month, patient A didn't take the drug for a while. On September 10th patient A had severe dental pain and presents to your pharmacy asking for a refill of his prescription. You, as the pharmacist, should:
    a. Refill the prescription as is
    b. Call the physician to obtain approval for filling
    c. Fill a 3-day supply
    d. Fill the prescription for cash
    e. Not fill the prescription

78. In which of the following situations would a faxed prescription from the physician's office to a retail pharmacy be allowed to serve as the original (i.e. no need to get an original hard copy of the prescription before dispensing)?

    I.   The practitioner prescribes the Schedule II controlled substances for a patient undergoing home infusion pain therapy.

    II. The practitioner prescribes the Schedule II controlled substances for a patient living in a long-term care facility.

    III. The practitioner prescribes the Schedule II controlled substances for a patient living in a hospice care facility.

    a. I only
    b. II only
    c. I and II only
    d. I and III only
    e. I, II, and III

79. What is true about dispensing controlled substance prescriptions in Kentucky?

    I. The Social Security number of the patient must be obtained before dispensing the controlled substance prescription.

    II. If the patient does not have a Social Security number, then the driver's license number of the patient must be obtained.

    III. If the patient does not have a Social Security number or a driver's license number, then the State Issued identification card is required to fill controlled substance prescription.

    a. I only
    b. II only
    c. I and II
    d. I, II, and III
    e. None of the above

80. A regular patient of yours comes to your pharmacy with the following prescription:

Methimazole 10mg
T1T PO QD # 30
5 refills

The patient tells you the prescption is written for his pet cat, Max. What information is required to be on the prescription? (select ALL that apply)
    a. Name of an animal
    b. Species of animal
    c. Full name and address of the owner of the animal
    d. DOB/ age of animal
    e. Diagnosis code for billing purposes

81. In the State of Kentucky, how much pseudoephedrine can a customer purchase?
    a. No more than 3.6 grams per purchase
    b. No more than 7.2 grams per purchase
    c. No more than 9.0 grams per month
    d. No more than 16.4 grams per 90 days
    e. No more than 26 grams per year

82. According to the Kentucky Revised Statutes: "A person is guilty of forgery of a prescription when, with intent to defraud, deceive, or injure another, he falsely makes, completes, or alters a written instrument which is or purports to be or which is calculated to become or to represent a prescription for a controlled substance when completed."

    What is the repercussion of a first offense of forgery of a prescription?
    a. Class A felony
    b. Class B felony
    c. Class C felony
    d. Class D felony
    e. A Misdemeanor

83. Which of the following is true regarding dispensing of Schedule V over-the-counter (OTC) products? (Select ALL that apply).
    a. The customer must be 21 years or older
    b. The sale should only be facilitated by a pharmacist-appointed designee
    c. Records of the sale must be maintained in a registry
    d. The medications should not be displayed in areas open to the public
    e. Codeine preparations must be combined with another non-codeine drug with different medicinal qualities

84. What medication does NOT require a medication guide to be included with its dispensing?
    a. Abilify
    b. Prozac
    c. Voltaren
    d. Synthroid
    e. Boniva

85. Patient Z is a 39-year-old female who presents to your pharmacy to fill an Adipex prescription written by her dentist. You as the pharmacist should:
    a. Not fill the prescription
    b. Fill the prescription as is
    c. Call the prescriber to obtain approval for filling the prescription
    d. Fill the Adipex only after filling out a KASPER report order form
    e. Not fill the prescription and ask the patient to obtain a new one

86. Choose the correct way for filing controlled substance prescriptions. (select ALL that apply)
    a. One file for CII, one file for III, IV, and V, one file for non-controlled
    b. One file for CII-CV, one file for non-controlled
    c. One file for CII, one file for CIII, IV, V and non-controlled
    d. One file for CII, one file for CII, IV, and V, one file for non-controlled, one file for OTC products
    e. All of the above

87. Which of the following statements is FALSE regarding home medical equipment in the State of Kentucky?
    a. It withstands repeated use
    b. It is not useful to a person without injury or illness
    c. It is used to serve a medical purpose
    d. It is appropriate for use at home and does not necessitate medical professional aid
    e. Home medical equipment companies do not require a license by the Board

88. You receive a prescription for oxycodone 5mg for a quantity of 120 tablets. Your patient's insurance only covers 90 tablets per fill. Your patient asks if you can bill the 90 tablets through their insurance plan but fill the remaining 30 tablets for the pharmacy's cash price. You tell them:
    a. No, this is not permitted under the Kentucky Controlled Substance Act
    b. No, this is not permitted under the FDA
    c. No, this requires approval from the prescriber
    d. Yes, as long as the partial fill is completed today
    e. Yes, as long as the partial fill is completed within 30 days of the date the prescription was written

89. A pharmacist sends an authorized reverse distributor controlled substances for disposal of outdated medications. The pharmacist must complete which of the following forms:
    a. DEA Form 222
    b. DEA Form 106
    c. DEA Form 41
    d. DEA Form 67
    e. DEA Form 218A

90. According to Kentucky State Pharmacy Law, what practitioners may prescribe Schedule II controlled substances in the course of their professional practices? (Select ALL that apply)
    a. Nurse practitioners
    b. Optometrists
    c. Physician's assistants
    d. Podiatrists
    e. Dentists

91. What is FALSE regarding medical gasses in the State of Kentucky?
    a. Medical gasses MUST be dispensed under a special pharmacy permit
    b. Medical gasses include nitrous oxide and oxygen
    c. Medical gasses require home health aide
    d. A special pharmacy permit is one that provides miscellaneous and specialized pharmacy service and functions
    e. Pharmacists in charge dispensing medical gasses should review pharmacy permits quarterly

92. A pharmacist receives a request for a prescription refill during a Governor-issued emergency. The prescription has no refill authorized, and the pharmacist is unable to obtain refill authorization from the prescriber due to the state of emergency. Under the condition, the pharmacist has authority to dispense a maximum:
    a. 72-hour supply
    b. 5-day supply
    c. 10-day supply
    d. 2-week supply
    e. 1-month supply

93. What is FALSE regarding situations where the Governor of Kentucky declares a state emergency?
    a. The Governor may issue an executive order for a period of up to thirty days giving pharmacists emergency authority
    b. A pharmacist may dispense up to a thirty-day emergency supply of medication
    c. A pharmacy may operate in an area not designated on the pharmacy permit
    d. A pharmacist may administer immunizations to children
    e. None of the above

94. The laminar air flow hood or other ISO class 5 environment must be certified:
    a. Weekly
    b. Monthly
    c. Quarterly
    d. Bi-Annually
    e. Annually

95. To whom can a confidential report be released to by a pharmacist?

    I.   The patient's next of kin

    II. The patient's prescriber

    III. The State Pharmacy Board

    IV. An insurance carrier

    a. I only
    b. I and II only
    c. I and IV only
    d. I, II, and IV
    e. I, II, III, and IV

96. Records of sales of Schedule V OTC products need to be maintained for:
    a. 6 months from the date of last transaction
    b. 12 months from the date of last transaction
    c. 1 year from the date of last transaction
    d. 2 years from the date of last transaction
    e. 5 years from the date of last transaction

97. Which drug is part of a class that is considered non-interchangeable by the Kentucky State Board of Pharmacy?
    a. Synthroid
    b. Methimazole
    c. Etodolac
    d. Albuterol
    e. Paxil

98. What security features MUST a prescription for a controlled substance contain? (select ALL that apply)
    a. A "Void" screen pattern across the entire prescription blank
    b. The prescription blank should not bear logos
    c. A watermark printed on the back of the prescription blank, only seen at a 45-degree angle
    d. If the prescription is photocopied, "Void" should appear across the prescription
    e. Only one prescription should be written per prescription blank

99. For what indications can a schedule II amphetamine or amphetamine-like controlled substance be used to treat? (select ALL that apply)
    a. Attention-deficit/hyperactivity disorder
    b. Narcolepsy
    c. Obesity (in combination with diet and exercise)
    d. Fatigue
    e. Resistant depressive disorder (in combination with antidepressants)

100. In the Commonwealth of Kentucky, on what date does pharmacy technician registration expire each year?
    a. February 28
    b. March 31
    c. June 30
    d. September 30
    e. December 31

Answer Index – Federal Questions

1 – b

The Pure Food and Drug Act of 1906 prohibited the distribution of food and drugs that were contaminated (adulterated) or not labeled consistently or correctly (misbranded).

2 – c

The Controlled Substance Ordering System (CSOS) is a secure, electronic program that can be used in place of a DEA Form 222 when ordering Schedule II controlled substances.

3 – d

The Drug Enforcement Administration (DEA) is part of the U.S. Department of Justice and is responsible for the federal CSA. The Controlled Substances Act is available online on the DEA website.

4 – d

The Orange Book (official name "Approved Drug Products with Therapeutic Equivalence Evaluations") is the primary source for determining therapeutic equivalency of drugs. The Purple Book lists biological products that are considered biosimilars and provides interchangeability evaluations for these products.

5 - b

When purchasing Schedule II controlled substances, the pharmacy (purchaser) will fill out a DEA Form 222 and submit it to the supplier. The supplier receives the original form. The purchaser is required to make a copy of the original DEA Form 222 for their records. This copy can be retained in paper or electronic form. Importantly, the purchaser does not have the option of keeping the original form.

6 – a

A DEA Form 106, titled "Report of Theft or Loss of Controlled Substances", is a form that must be filled out and submitted to the DEA upon discovery of theft or significant loss of controlled substances. There is a section of the DEA form 106 that allows the user to list out the controlled substances and quantities that were stolen or lost. Submitting a DEA form 106 formally documents the situation and the pharmacy should retain a copy for their records. The DEA must also immediately be contacted by phone, fax, or brief written message to alert them of the situation. The local authorities should also be alerted.

7 – b

An IND must be submitted and approved by the FDA before a drug can be tested in humans. This is used for drugs that have not been marketed in the U.S. and for the purpose of investigation in clinical trials. The FDA has 30 days to decide if the drug is suitable for testing after the submission of the application. After approval, the sponsor that submitted the application can start testing.

8 – b

Clinical trials for an investigational new drug are generally conducted in four phases: Phase I, Phase II, Phase III, and Phase IV. Each phase is designed to gather different information. There is not a Phase V.

- Phase I clinical trials are used to assess the drug properties, such as pharmacokinetics and adverse effects. These initial trials are conducted in a small group of healthy participants.

- Phase II clinical trials focus on assessing efficacy of a drug compared to a standard treatment or placebo.

- Phase III clinical trials are used to provide a more comprehensive understanding of the potential benefits and risks of a drug. The sample population is larger in Phase III.

- Phase IV clinical trials are post-marketing surveillance trials to collect information about problems or adverse effects with the drug after it is marketed.

9 – a

The Prescription Drug Marketing Act (PDMA) of 1987 involves several laws regarding prescription drugs. Primarily, it regulates the storage, distribution, and resale of drug samples. It enforces recordkeeping requirements for prescription drug samples. The PDMA also prohibits hospitals and other health care entities from reselling their drugs to other businesses. This is because hospitals usually obtain drugs at a special rate. Finally, it regulates state licensing of wholesalers.

10 – a

A Prior Approval Supplement (older term Supplemental New Drug Application) is submitted to the FDA when a manufacturer wants to change anything related to the location or process of manufacturing. This includes the location of manufacturing, procedures, drug synthesis, packaging, etc.

11 – c

The FDA has developed four distinct processes to speed up the process of making drugs available as fast as possible. The four approaches are:

- Fast track

- Breakthrough therapy

- Accelerated approval

- Priority review

Fast track is an expedited review process intended for drugs that treat serious conditions and fill an unmet medical need. Breakthrough therapy is a process designed to expedite the development and review of drugs which may demonstrate substantial improvement over available therapy. Accelerated approval is for drugs with long-term endpoints that are hard to measure during clinical trials, such as a decrease in mortality or increase in survival. These drugs are approved based on a surrogate endpoint. Finally, priority review designation means the FDA's goal is to take action on the application within six months. "Instant approval" is not an FDA process.

12 - d

Schedule II controlled substances can be transferred in all of the given scenarios except for a researcher transferring Schedule II controlled substances to a pharmacy to be dispensed to patients. Researchers must be authorized to conduct research with Schedule II controlled substances. Researchers may transfer Schedule II controlled substances to another authorized researcher for the purpose of research. Researchers may not transfer Schedule II controlled substances to a pharmacy.

13 – b

Once a pharmacy has filled and dispensed a medication, the prescription is legally owned by the pharmacy and the original prescription can't be returned to the patient. However, it is acceptable to make a copy for the patient or the prescriber if needed.

The prescription can be transferred to another pharmacy (if legal depending on the schedule and number of refills remaining), but the pharmacy that originally filled the prescription must retain the original copy.

14 – b

Adulteration involves the integrity and composition of a product. If the composition or integrity of a drug is compromised, then the drug is considered adulterated. Some examples of adulteration include:

- A drug contains a decomposed substance

- A drug that is not manufactured under required manufacturing standards

- A drug that is stored in unsanitary conditions

- A substance of the drug container leaches into the drug itself

- A drug that is not pure or contains less than the listed amount of active ingredient

- A drug that contains an unapproved color additive

15 – a

The Food, Drug, and Cosmetic Act (FDCA) requires all new drugs to be proven safe for their labeled use before they can be marketed to patients. This Act was passed in 1938 after a drug called elixir sulfanilamide caused mass poisonings and over a hundred deaths in the United States.

16 – e

The Good Manufacturing Practice (GMP) is a set of regulations that determines minimum standards for pharmaceutical manufacturing in the U.S. The purpose of GMP is to uphold the safety and quality of drug products.

17 – c

National Drug Codes (NDCs) are drug identification numbers that are unique to each drug manufactured. The NDC contains 3 sets of numbers:

1) The first set is either a 4- or 5-digit number and represents the manufacturer.

2) The second set is a 4-digit number that represents the identity of the drug.

3) The third set is a 2-digit number that is the product package size, such as the bottle count, blister packs, etc.

Let's say we have levothyroxine 50 mcg that is supplied as a 100-count bottle and a 500-count bottle from the same manufacturer. The NDC code will be the same except for the last 2 numbers because the bottle count sizes are different.

18 – d

Pentobarbital is a Schedule II controlled substance. It is a barbiturate. Schedule II controlled substances include, but are not limited to: opiates and opioids, amphetamines and dextroamphetamine salts, pentobarbital, secobarbital, and phencyclidine. Mescaline is a Schedule I controlled substance. Butabarbital is a Schedule III controlled substance. Modafinil is a Schedule IV controlled substance. Finally, buprenorphine is a Schedule III controlled substance.

19 – d

On a federal level, Schedule III and IV controlled substances can be filled up to 5 times in a 6-month period from the date the prescription was written. Some states also apply this refill rule to Schedule V controlled substances.

20 – d

No directions for administration are necessary for oral drug products. However, if drugs are not for oral use, then the specific route(s) of administration must be stated.

Label requirements for the manufacturer container include: name and address of the manufacturer/packer/distributor, name of drug or product, net quantity packaged, weights of each active ingredient, route(s) of administration for non-oral medications, manufacturer control or lot number, expiration date, special storage instructions if applicable, and the federal legend (e.g. "Rx only").

21 – c

A water-containing oral formulation made from commercially available drug products has a maximum BUD of 14 days when stored in the refrigerator. Non-aqueous formulations have a maximum BUD of 6 months. Water-containing topical/dermals, mucosal liquids, and semisolid formulations have a maximum beyond-use date of 30 days. Drugs or chemicals that are known to be labile to decomposition will require shorter BUDs. Finally, the BUD cannot exceed the expiration date of the active pharmaceutical ingredient (API) or any other component in the product.

22 – d

According to the Code of Federal Regulations, mid-level practitioners are defined as individual practitioners other than physicians, dentists, veterinarians, or podiatrists. Mid-level practitioners include, but are not limited to: nurse practitioners, nurse midwives, nurse anesthetists, clinical nurse specialists, physician assistants, optometrists, homeopathic physicians, registered pharmacists, and certified chiropractors.

23 – a, d, e

DME is made for long-term use and must be able to withstand repeated use, be primarily for a medical purpose, and be appropriate for home use. It includes many different types of devices for individuals with a variety of conditions. Some examples of durable medical equipment include wheelchairs, crutches, canes, oxygen, ventilators, and hospital beds.

24 – c

The Controlled Substances Registrant Protection Act (CSRPA) of 1984 was enacted to protect DEA registrants against certain crimes. It provides federal investigation in cases where any of the following are met:

- The cost to replace the stolen controlled substances is $500 or more

- An employee obtains significant injury or was killed

- Interstate or foreign commerce was involved in the execution of the crime.

The perpetrator(s) may be subject to fines and/or imprisonment. Theft occurring during drug transport to the pharmacy is not one of the conditions.

25 – e

Omnibus Budget Reconciliation Act of 1990 (commonly known as OBRA 90) set the requirement that patients must be offered counseling on the medications. Patients have the right to refuse this counseling, but counseling must at least be offered.

26 – a

Isotretinoin is an oral medication used to treat severe acne. Taking isotretinoin during pregnancy can cause birth defects, therefore this drug is highly regulated through a REMS program.

The REMS program for isotretinoin is called iPLEDGE. Under iPLEDGE:

- Only doctors registered with iPLEDGE may prescribe isotretinoin

- Only patients registered with iPLEDGE may receive isotretinoin

- Only pharmacies registered with iPLEDGE may dispense isotretinoin.

- Patients may receive no more than a 30-day supply at a time.

- No refills are allowed on prescriptions for isotretinoin.

- Female patients who can get pregnant must use 2 separate methods of effective birth control 1 month before, while taking, and for 1 month after taking isotretinoin.

- Female patients who can get pregnant must take a pregnancy test every month.

27 – b

Compounded drugs cannot be compounded, provided, or sold to other pharmacies or third parties. Compounded drugs cannot be commercially available, must meet national standards, must be a reasonable quantity for current or anticipated prescriptions, and distribution cannot be more than 5% of total prescriptions filled by the pharmacy per year. Drugs that have been removed from the market are also not allowed to be used in compounding. Compounding may be an option to customize medications based upon a doctor's prescription. For example, compounding can customize a drug strength, remove an allergic component, flavor a medication, and change the dosage form.

28 – b

A DEA Form 222 or an electronically equivalent program is necessary in order to purchase or transfer Schedule II controlled substances.

29 – d

The Schedule II controlled substance prescription can be mailed to the patient. Controlled substances used to not be able to be mailed, but this is no longer the case. The package must contain an inner package with the prescription and appropriate labeling, but must be placed in a plain outer container. The outside package cannot contain information about the contents of the package.

30 – c

Narrow therapeutic index drugs are drugs where small differences in the dose or blood concentration may lead to serious therapeutic failures or adverse reactions. These drugs require careful titration or patient monitoring for safe and effective use. They are permitted to be prescribed. Some drugs with a narrow therapeutic index are: warfarin, levothyroxine, digoxin, lithium carbonate, phenytoin, and cyclosporine. Additionally, the FDA recommends that potency of the drug have a variability limit of 90% to 105% when the drugs are manufactured.

31 – a

The Poison Prevention Packaging Act (PPPA) set the requirement that prescription drugs, non-prescription drugs, and hazardous household products must have a child-resistant closure. The purpose was to protect children less than 5 years old from accidental poisoning from accidental ingestion or exposure. Patients may ask to not have safety caps on their medications, especially if they have conditions such as arthritis that make it difficult for them to open up the containers. There are also several prescription drugs that are exempt from PPPA, such as nitroglycerin sublingual tablets, oral contraceptive in mnemonic dispenser package, isosorbide dinitrate sublingual and chewable forms, and more.

32 – b

A Class II drug recall occurs when the product may cause temporary or medically reversible adverse effects, but the probability of serious adverse effects is remote.

33 – b

Phase 1 clinical trials are conducted in a small group of healthy participants without the disease condition. Typically the study size is around 20–80 people. The goal of the Phase 1 clinical trial is to study the properties of the drug and determine safety. Sometimes the Phase 1 clinical trial can include participants with the disease condition, but this is not as common.

Phase 2 clinical trials are conducted in a larger size group of 100 or more people, and these participants have the disease condition. Phase 2 clinical trials study the effectiveness of the drug.

Phase 3 clinical trials are conducted in a larger group of hundreds or thousands of participants who have the disease condition. The drug's safety, efficacy, and dosing are further studied. If a drug passes the Phase 3 study, then it can be approved by the FDA.

Finally, Phase 4 clinical trials are conducted after the drug is approved and looks at the safety and efficacy of the drug long-term, also called post-marketing surveillance.

34 – b

A drug product manufactured in the U.S., sent out to a foreign country, and then re-imported back to the U.S. is only legal if it is done by the original manufacturer. Re-importation is permitted by the original manufacturer if the purpose is for emergency medical care. Otherwise, re-importation of drugs is not permitted. As some background information, some consumers will want to engage in drug re-importation because drugs may be sold at a lower price outside of the United States. Re-importation is a potential way to obtain access to another country's lower drug prices, particularly from Canada and Mexico.

35 – e

The Kefauver-Harris Amendment requires that manufacturers provide proof of the effectiveness and safety of their drugs before these drugs can be approved. This was the first "proof-of-efficacy" requirement. The situation that prompted this amendment was the use of thalidomide in Europe that was marketed as a sedative-hypnotic drug that could be used during pregnancy, but it caused serious birth defects. Before the Kefauver-Harris Amendment, the Food, Drug, and Cosmetic Act (FDCA) of 1939 required drugs be proven safe before being marketed.

36 – c

Pharmacies will use DEA Form 224 to register with the DEA to possess and dispense controlled substances. DEA Form 106 is to report theft or loss of controlled substances. DEA Form 222 to order and transfer Schedule I and II controlled substances. DEA Form 225 is used by manufacturers, distributors, importers, exporters, and researchers to register to conduct business with controlled substances. DEA Form 363 is used by Narcotic Treatment Programs to register to conduct business with controlled substances.

37 – c

Under the Drug Supply Chain Security Act, manufacturers are required to provide a transaction report (pedigree) for each product sold. Pharmacies are required to receive this information and pass it along if they further distribute the product. This allows the drugs to be tracked. The transaction report includes 3 parts, also known informally as the "3 T's": Transaction information, Transaction history, and Transaction statement.

38 – a

Drug recalls are classified as Class I, II, or III, from most severe to least severe. A Class I recall is when a product may cause serious adverse health issues or death. A Class II recall is when a product has a low likelihood of causing serious adverse effects, but may cause some temporary or reversible adverse effects. A Class III recall is when a product is not likely to cause adverse health consequences.

39 – c

The Safe Medical Device Act (SMDA) of 1990 requires health care facilities to report death or injuries caused by or suspected to have been caused by a medical device to the FDA or the manufacturer. The goal is to quickly inform the FDA on the issue so the product can be tracked and potentially recalled for safety reasons. Some examples of medical devices that could be reported are: defibrillators, shunts, lab reagents, pulse oximeters, glucose meters, infusion pumps, wheelchairs, ventilator breathing circuits, needles, catheters, and more.

40 – c

Misbranding is inaccurate labeling on the drug container. If information is missing, inaccurate, or untrue, this is considered misbranding. Examples of misbranding include: false or misleading information, unreadable material, omitting a medication guide, inadequate directions or warnings, omitting required information, etc.

41 – b

Methadone is used for both the treatment of pain (i.e. as an analgesic) and in the detoxification and maintenance of narcotic addiction in patients registered in a narcotic treatment program. While a retail pharmacy may stock methadone, methadone can only be dispensed as an analgesic. Methadone can only be dispensed for the maintenance or detoxification of addicts when it is provided through a registered narcotic treatment center. It can be provided through one of these centers for either short-term detoxification (up to 30 days), or long-term detoxification (30–180 days).

42 – c

A drug (or biologic) is considered to be an orphan drug if it is intended to treat a rare disease or condition that impacts fewer than 200,000 people in the U.S. Sometimes, an orphan drug designation can be given to drugs citing a cost recovery provision, which is if the cost of research and development of the drug is not reasonably expected to be regained by sales of the drug.

43 – b

Several ingredients such as FD&C Yellow No. 5, aspartame, wintergreen oil, mineral oil, salicylates, sulfites, Ipecac syrup, and alcohol have special labeling requirements under federal regulations. FD&C Yellow No. 5, also called tartrazine, is a color additive that may cause an allergic reaction (itching and hives) in some people. Therefore, a product that contains FD&C Yellow No. 5 must identify so on the label.

44 – e

Normally, a faxed prescription for a Schedule II controlled substance cannot be accepted. However, there are 3 exceptions. Prescriptions for Schedule II controlled substances can be faxed and serve as the original prescription for patients residing in a long-term care facility, enrolled in hospice, or if the drug is to be compounded for direct administration by parenteral, intravenous, intramuscular, subcutaneous, or intraspinal infusion (which includes home infusion therapy).

45 – b

The FDA Adverse Event Reporting System (FAERS) is a database where adverse events from medications can be voluntarily reported. This provides post-marketing safety surveillance on medications.

Meanwhile, the VAERS stands for the Vaccine Adverse Event Reporting System, which is a national vaccine safety surveillance program run by the CDC and FDA.

ERSA, MAERS, and AERS are not drug-related reporting systems.

46 – c

A prescription for a Schedule II controlled substance can be called in orally to be dispensed in an emergency situation. The prescription should be immediately written down by the pharmacist. The quantity should only be enough to adequately cover the emergency period. The pharmacy needs to receive a hard copy prescription from the prescriber within 7 days after authorizing the emergency dispensing. This must also have the words "authorization for emergency dispensing" on the prescription and the date of the oral order written on the front. Prescriptions postmarked within the 7 day period are acceptable. If the prescription is not received in a timely manner, this should be reported to the DEA.

47 – b

The Purple Book contains information related to biological products and information regarding interchangeable biological products. The Orange Book provides information regarding therapeutic equivalence between drugs (excluding biologics). The Red Book is used for drug pricing and packaging information. The Pink Book contains information related to immunizations and vaccine-preventable diseases, as well as information on vaccine safety. Information and recommendation related to international travel (vaccines, diseases, information of other health risks) can be bound in the Yellow Book.

48 – e

An exact count must be made on controlled substances if it is a Schedule I or II controlled substance, if it is a controlled substance where the bottle contains more than 1000 tablets or capsules, and if the containers are sealed or unopened. Sealed or unopened containers do not need to be opened and counted, but the number marked as the container quantity must be used as an exact count.

49 – b

The U.S. Attorney General, as head of the Justice Department (which the Drug Enforcement Administration is under), may add, delete, or reschedule substances. A scientific and medical recommendation from the Food and Drug Administration is included in the decision.

50 – c

A full NDA must be submitted to the FDA when a manufacturer wants to request reclassification of a current prescription-only drug to be an over-the-counter drug. This is just one method of requesting reclassification, as there are four different methods. Another method is the FDA granting an exemption if determining prescription-only status is not necessary for the safety and protection of the public. A third method is filing a supplement to the original NDA (a "supplemental NDA") for review of the drug's safety and adverse events. The last method is if the Nonprescription Drug Advisory Committee recommends the ingredient contained in the drug be converted to a non-prescription status.

An ANDA is an application for the potential approval of a generic drug product. Both EIND and IND are applications regarding the development of a new drug. A marketed new drug application is not an existing type of application.

51 – a

In order to verify a DEA number, use the following process:

1) Add together the first, third, and fifth numbers.

2) Add together the second, fourth, and sixth numbers. Multiply this number by two.

3) Add the numbers together from steps 1 and 2. The last digit of the number you get from step 3 is the last number of the DEA number.

Using the DEA number BS5927683, the process would be:

1) $5 + 2 + 6 = 13$

2) $(9 + 7 + 8) \times 2 = (24) \times 2 = 48$

3) $13 + 48 = 61 \rightarrow$ Since the last digit is 1, the DEA should end in 1, not 3.

52 – d

Dentists must prescribe within their scope of practice. Accordingly, prescriptions written by a dentist must treat a disease of the mouth, discomfort in the mouth, or to facilitate a dental procedure. Atorvastatin is used to lower cholesterol. Other health professions, such as optometrists and veterinarians, must also prescribe within their scope of practice.

53 – e

A DEA Form 222 must be signed and dated by the person authorized to sign the pharmacy's DEA registration. This means that only the pharmacist who signed the most recent application for renewal of the pharmacy's DEA registration may sign a DEA Form 222. Additionally, that pharmacist may authorize others to sign a DEA Form 222 by granting a power of attorney. A power of attorney must be signed by the registrant (name of person granting the power), the person to whom the power of attorney is being granted, and two witnesses.

54 – a

OTC drug advertising is regulated by the Federal Trade Commission (FTC). On the other hand, prescription drug advertising is regulated by the Food and Drug Administration (FDA).

55 – c

A pharmacy may keep shipping and financial data for controlled substances at a central location other than the registered location after notifying the nearest DEA Diversion Field Office. Executed DEA form 222 orders, controlled substance prescriptions, and controlled substance inventories must be kept at the pharmacy location that is registered with the DEA, and cannot be kept at a central location.

56 – c

Schedule III controlled substances have less potential for abuse than Schedule I or II drugs, and they have a currently accepted medical use in the U.S. Codeine by itself is classified under Schedule II, but in combination with acetaminophen it is a Schedule III drug.

57 – e

HIPAA permits the use of protected health information (PHI) for treatment purposes. Medical information can be shared to persons involved in the patient's care without written or verbal consent.

58 – b

The Federal Transfer Warning ("Caution: Federal law prohibits the transfer of this drug to any person other than the patient for whom it was prescribed") is required on the label of Schedule II–IV controlled substances when dispensed to a patient. Most pharmacies comply with this requirement by including this warning on all prescription labels. However, it is not legally required on prescription labels for Schedule V controlled substances and non-controlled prescriptions.

59 – a

Outsourcing facilities, also known as 503B facilities, are permitted to compound sterile products without receiving patient-specific prescriptions or medication orders. They are regulated by the FDA and subject to current good manufacturing practices. Compounded products must be distributed within a health care setting or dispensed directly to a patient or prescriber, and may not be sold or transferred to a wholesaler for redistribution.

A pharmacy that registers as an outsourcing facility would therefore be able to compound sterile products without receiving patient-specific prescriptions.

60 – a, b, d

There are three different options for filing paper prescriptions under federal law. The first option is to separate prescription records into 3 buckets:

1) Schedule II

2) Schedule III–V

3) Non-controlled

The second option is filing into 2 buckets:

1) Schedule II

2) Schedule III–V and non-controlled together, but marking Schedule III–V with a red "C"

The third option is filing into 2 buckets:

1) Schedule II–V, but marking Schedule III–V with a red "C"

2) Non-controlled

Note that if a state has stricter state laws, those should be followed. Additionally, a pharmacy has the option of storing prescription files electronically. Electronic prescription files must be readily retrievable.

61 – d

The USP Chapter <797> describes the requirements of sterile compounded preparations, including responsibilities of compounding personnel, training, facilities, environmental monitoring, and storage and testing. USP Chapter <795> covers nonsterile compounding, and USP Chapter <800> describes safe handling of hazardous drugs. USP <503A> and USP <503B> do not exist as USP chapters; however, the terms 503A and 503B are used to designate compounding pharmacies.

62 – b, c, d

Every person or firm that manufactures, distributes, or dispenses any controlled substance must register with the DEA. However, patients who receive controlled substance prescriptions and pharmacists working in a pharmacy are exempt from DEA registration requirements. Therefore, pharmacists do not need to have a DEA number to dispense controlled substances.

63 – b

Clozapine is associated with severe neutropenia, which can lead to severe infections. Prescribers are required to be certified in the clozapine REMS program before prescribing clozapine. Pharmacies are also required to be certified in the clozapine REMS program to dispense clozapine.

64 – c

A DEA Form 41 is used to document the destruction of controlled substances. More commonly, a pharmacy will transfer controlled substances to an authorized reverse distributor for destruction. The reverse distributor then fills out DEA Form 41 to document the destruction of controlled substances.

65 – b

The Federal Anti-Tampering Act requires tamper-evident packaging of many over-the-counter products and cosmetics to avoid contamination issues and limit access. If the items were tampered with, it would be evident due to the packaging of these products. For example, some products have a tamper-evident closure cap, tamper-evident liner, and tamper-evident tape. The Act was passed in response to the Tylenol poisoning deaths in Chicago in 1982, where the Tylenol capsules were contaminated with cyanide.

66 – a

Schedule I controlled substances include drugs that have a high potential for abuse and severe potential for dependence, with no currently accepted medical use in the U.S. This includes heroin, lysergic acid diethylamide (LSD), mescaline, and methaqualone, among others.

67 – c

Manufacturer's containers of OTC medications are required to display the following information: identity of the product (active ingredient), inactive ingredient(s), purpose, use(s), warnings, directions, storage information.

Other information that is not required, but may be included: net quantity of contents, name and address of the manufacturer/ packager/distributor, lot number or batch code, expiration date, and instructions for what to do if an overdose occurs.

While the Poison Control Center phone number is included on some OTC medications, it is not required by federal law.

68 – b

Patient Package Inserts (PPIs) must be provided to patients in acute-care hospitals or long-term care facilities prior to the first administration and every 30 days thereafter. They are required for oral contraceptives and estrogen-containing products.

69 – c

DEA registration permits pharmacies, manufacturers, distributors, importers, exporters, and researchers to possess controlled substances. A DEA registration is valid for 36 months. Registrants will receive renewal notification approximately 60 days prior to the DEA registration expiration date.

70 – c

For recordkeeping requirements, executed copies of DEA Form 222 must be maintained separately from all other records. If a pharmacy stores these forms electronically, then the electronic records are deemed separate if such copies are readily retrievable from all other electronic records. A defective DEA Form 222 cannot be corrected and needs to be replaced by a new form. Finally, when filling out the DEA Form 222, only 1 item may be entered on each numbered line.

71 – e

Under the Health Insurance Portability and Accountability Act (HIPAA) Privacy Rule, a communication is not considered "marketing" if it is made for the treatment of the individual. Therefore, refill reminders for currently prescribed medications (or one that has not lapsed for more than 90 days) are not considered marketing. Therefore, offering this service is not a HIPAA violation. Patients may be charged for this service as long as any payment made to the pharmacy is reasonable and related to the pharmacy's cost of making the communication. Mailed refill reminders are valid, as well as electronic refill reminders.

As a note, the HIPAA Privacy Rule defines marketing as making "a communication about a product or service that encourages recipients of the communication to purchase or use the product or service." An entity would need to receive authorization from the patient to send out marketing communications.

72 – d

Manufacturer's expiration dates may be expressed as a day, month, and year, or as just a month and year. If it is written as only month and year, the drug expires on the last day of the listed month. The drug is safe to use on the expiration date, but not after.

73 – c

A prospective DUR consists of reviewing a prescription for adverse effects, therapeutic duplication, drug-disease interactions and contraindications, drug dosing and regimen, drug allergies, clinical misuse or abuse, drug interactions, medication appropriateness, overutilization, underutilization, and pregnancy alerts. Ensuring compliance with prescription labeling is not part of the prospective DUR.

74 – a

The purpose of the Federal Hazardous Substances Act (FHSA) is to protect consumers from hazardous or toxic substances. The FHSA requires precautionary labeling on the immediate container of hazardous household products, which includes certain OTC medications. Medication packages would include the statement, "Keep out of the reach of children." Depending on the hazardous substance, additional warnings and statements, such as "handle with gloves" or "harmful if swallowed", may be required. The warning "Keep out of the reach of children" applies to OTC drugs and not FDA-regulated drugs.

75 – c

The 5% rule states that a pharmacy does not have to register with the DEA as a distributor if the total quantity of controlled substances distributed during a 12-month period does not exceed 5% of the total quantity of all controlled substances dispensed and distributed during that period.

76 – d

The Occupational and Safety Health Administration (OSHA) requires that employers meet the Hazardous Communication Standard. This includes having a Hazardous Communication Plan, which lists hazardous chemicals in the workplace, and ensuring that all such products are appropriately labeled and have a Safety Data Sheet. Workers must be trained on the hazards of chemicals, appropriate protective measures, and where to find more information. The purpose of OSHA is to protect employees, which is separate from laws intended to protect consumers and patients.

77 – b

The Consumer Product Safety Commission administers the Poison Prevention Packaging Act (PPPA). This Act requires child-resistant containers for all prescriptions and certain non-prescription drugs, unless there is an exemption for a specific drug or circumstance.

78 – d

Bulk compounding of products in order to sell them to other pharmacies is considered "manufacturing," which is regulated by the FDA. Note that for manufacturing, a patient-specific prescription is not required. So, in this case, since there is not a patient-specific prescription involved, the mass production of ibuprofen suppositories is considered manufacturing. On the other hand, "compounding" is typically regulated by state boards of pharmacy and is limited to compounding prescriptions for individual patients pursuant to a prescription.

79 – e

The Prescription Drug Marketing Act bans most pharmacies from purchasing, trading, selling, or possessing prescription drug samples. The only exception is for pharmacies that are owned by a charitable organization or by a city, state, or county government and that are part of a health care entity providing care to indigent or low-income patients at no or reduced cost. In this case, samples may only be provided at no cost to the patients.

80 – e

DEA Form 222 is used to transfer and order Schedule II controlled substances. The DEA used to allow this form to be faxed, but not anymore. A DEA Form 224 is needed for a pharmacy to dispense controlled substances. Schedule III–V controlled substances may be ordered through normal ordering processes from wholesalers or manufacturers, but must be documented by the pharmacy with an invoice upon receipt. The common term used for ordering Schedule III–V controlled substances is using an "invoice."

81 – d

Manufacturers and packagers of over-the-counter drugs for sale at retail must package products in tamper-evident packaging, with some exceptions. The exceptions are dermatological, dentifrice, insulin, or lozenge products.

82 – c

A pharmacist may not change the following items on a Schedule II controlled substance prescription: name of the patient, name of the drug, and the name of the prescriber. All other information, including quantity, directions for use, drug strength, and dosage form, may be changed with the verbal permission of the prescriber as long as the change is documented on the prescription.

83 – e

Patients have a right to obtain a copy of their protected health information. Pharmacies must comply with such a request within 30 days. If there is a delay, the patient must be notified of the reason for delay and the pharmacy may extend the time by no more than 30 additional days. Normally, pharmacies are able to give a copy of the prescription record the day of the request.

84 - b

Thalidomide is an immunomodulatory agent as well as a chemotherapy drug. Thalidomide causes a high frequency of birth defects in pregnant females. Babies were born with missing or deformed arms and legs. Therefore, the REMS program was developed to ensure safe use and monitoring of thalidomide.

85 – c

The Kefauver-Harris Amendment of 1962 is more commonly known as the "Drug Efficacy Amendment." It requires new drugs to be proven as safe and effective before they are approved. It also allows the FDA to establish good drug manufacturing practices and gives the FDA jurisdiction over prescription drug advertising, which must include accurate information about side effects. It also controls the marketing of generic drugs to keep them from being sold as expensive medications under new trade names.

86 – c

Anabolic steroids are classified as Schedule III controlled substances under federal law. An example of an anabolic steroid is testosterone.

87 – d

The Durham-Humphrey Amendment created two separate categories of drugs, prescription (legend) and over-the-counter (OTC). Prescription drugs require a prescription and must be dispensed under medical supervision. OTC drugs can be obtained without a prescription and do not require medical supervision.

88 – d

Generic bioequivalence information is found in the FDA Orange Book. A two-letter coding system indicates equivalency, with the first letter being key. Codes that start with the letter A indicate that the FDA considers the drug products to be pharmaceutically and therapeutically equivalent. Codes that start with the letter B indicate that the FDA does not consider the products to be equivalent.

The second letter of the code typically indicates the dosage form (for example, a code of AT would indicate that two topical products are equivalent).

Products with known or potential equivalency issues, but for which adequate scientific evidence exists to establish bioequivalence, are given a code of AB.

89 – a, b, d

DEA registration is not required for an agent or employee of any registered manufacturer, distributor, or dispenser if acting in the usual course of business. This includes pharmacists working at pharmacies and nurses working in a hospital or physician's office. Patients who possess controlled substances for a lawful purpose are not required to register with the DEA.

Providers must register with the DEA unless practicing under the registration of a hospital or other institution. Each pharmacy must have its own DEA registration to dispense controlled substances.

90 – d

A product is considered adulterated if its strength or quality differs from what it represents (this is not the only criteria for adulteration, but one example). A product is misbranded if the labeling is false or misleading. If a drug product's strength is less than what is represented on the label, then the drug product is considered both adulterated and misbranded.

91 – d

Patients may request easy-open containers (containers that are not child-resistant) for any prescription. A provider may also make this request on a patient's behalf (written or verbal), but can only do so for one individual prescription. Only a patient can issue a blanket request for easy-open containers on all future prescriptions. There is not a legal requirement for documentation of easy-open container requests, but it is good practice for a pharmacist to have documentation in case an issue arises.

92 – c

Risk Evaluation and Mitigation Strategies (REMS) are strategies to manage a known or potential serious risk associated with a drug. A REMS program does not have anything to do with the affordability of drugs.

93 – c

Federal regulations require a warning on aspirin and other salicylate products, including a risk of Reye's syndrome in children. An example warning statement is: "Keep out of reach of children. In case of overdose, get medical help or contact a Poison Control Center right away." Containers of chewable 81mg (1.25 grain) aspirin may not contain more than 36 tablets in order to reduce the risk of accidental poisoning in children. In other words, if a child were to open a bottle of aspirin and ingest all 36 tablets, 36 tablets would generally be considered a non-toxic amount.

94 – b

DEA Registration numbers begin with two letters. The first letter indicates practitioner status, in which "M" is the designation for mid-level practitioners. The second letter typically indicates the first letter of the practitioner's last name, the first letter of the pharmacy name, or the first letter of the hospital name. To verify the DEA registration number, first add together the 1st, 3rd, and 5th digit. Then add together the 2nd, 4th, and 6th digit, and multiply this number by two. Add these two numbers together. The last digit (in the ones place) of the sum of these two numbers should match the last number of the DEA Registration number.

Check each of the five choices. For the second choice (MT1200980):

1) $1 + 0 + 9 = 10$

2) $2 + 0 + 8 = 10$; $10 \times 2 = 20$

3) $10 + 20 = 30$

The last digit of 30 is 0, so 0 must be the last digit of the DEA number: MT1200980.

95 – a, b, d

The FDA requires Medication Guides be issued with certain prescription drugs and biologics if they determine the drug has serious risks relative to benefits, when patient adherence is crucial to the effectiveness of the drug, when there is a known serious side effect, and when providing information can prevent serious adverse effects. Medication guides do not replace pharmacist counseling. A patient also does not need to be in a nursing home to receive a medication guide. Some drugs which require a guide be dispensed with each fill are: aripiprazole, amphetamine/dextroamphetamine, fentanyl, testosterone, citalopram, ciprofloxacin, amiodarone, duloxetine, adalimumab, and more.

96 – a, b, c

An NDC number is a numeric, 3-segment code that identifies a drug by manufacturer (first 4 or 5 numbers), specific drug (next 4 numbers), and package (last 2 numbers). NDC numbers are unique to each drug and serve as a universal product identifier for drugs. The expiration date information is not included in the NDC number. By law, the FDA does not require that drug manufacturers include NDC numbers on labels, but it is highly recommended.

NDC numbers are published in an NDC Directory by the FDA. The labeler is responsible for the content of the NDC entry, not the FDA. Therefore, inclusion of information in the NDC directory doesn't mean that the FDA has verified the information. Additionally, assignment of an NDC number does not mean the drug has been approved by the FDA.

97 – a, b, e

Several drugs are exempt from the child-resistant container packaging requirement. Some examples include sublingual nitroglycerin tablets, methylprednisolone tablets containing no more than 84mg per package, preparations in aerosol containers intended for inhalation, and more. Effervescent aspirin or acetaminophen tablets are exempt, but non-effervescent tablets are not. Packages of prednisone tablets are only exempt if they contain less than 105mg per package.

98 – b

Prescription records are required to be kept for a minimum of 2 years based on federal law. However, if there are stricter state laws, those should be followed. For example, if a state requires prescription records to be maintained for 5 years, then prescription records must be maintained for at least 5 years because it is stricter than 2 years.

99 – b, c, e

The Health Information Technology for Economic and Clinical Health Act (HITECH Act) promotes health information technology to advance healthcare, specifically advancing the use of electronic health records. The HIPAA Breach Notification Rule is a part of this Act. It requires entities to notify affected individuals without unreasonable delay, and in no case later than 60 days following the discovery of a breach of unsecured protected health information. Breaches of 500 or more records also need to be reported to the U.S. Department of Health and Human Services (HHS) within 60 days of the discovery of the breach, and smaller breaches within 60 days of the end of the calendar year in which the breach occurred. In addition to reporting the breach to the HHS, a notice of a breach of 500 or more records must be provided to prominent media outlets serving the state or jurisdiction affected by the breach.

100 – b

CMS regulations require a consultant pharmacist to perform a Drug Regimen Review for long-term care patients at least once a month.

Answer Index – Kentucky Questions

1 – c

A pharmacy which has mailed or shipped a controlled substance to a location in Kentucky and learns that the mailing or shipment did not arrive must within three business days report that nonreceipt to the Department of Kentucky State Police and, if applicable, the United States Postal Inspection Service.

2 – c

Each out of state pharmacy during its regular hours of operation, but not less than 6 days per week and for a minimum of forty hours per week, provide a toll-free telephone service directly to the pharmacist in charge of the out of state pharmacy and available to both the patient and each licensed and practicing in-state pharmacist for the purpose of facilitating communication between the patient and the Kentucky pharmacist with access to the patient's prescription records.

3 – c

Any pharmacy within the Commonwealth that dispenses more than 25% of its total prescription volume as a result of an original prescription order received or solicited by use of the Internet, including but not limited to electronic mail, shall, prior to obtaining a permit, receive and display in every medium in which it advertises itself a seal of approval for the National Association of Boards of Pharmacy certifying that it is a Verified Internet Pharmacy Practice Site (VIPPS) or a seal certifying approval of a substantially similar program approved by the Kentucky Board of Pharmacy.

VIPPS, or any other substantially similar program approved by the Kentucky Board of Pharmacy, accreditation shall be maintained and remain current.

Any pharmacy within the Commonwealth doing business by use of the Internet must certify the percentage of its annual business conducted via the Internet and submit such supporting documentation as requested by the Board, and in a form or application required by the Board, when it applies for permit or renewal.

4 – e

Every applicant for licensure as a pharmacist must be:

- Not less than eighteen (18) years of age

- Of good mental health and moral character

- A graduate of a school or college of pharmacy program approved by the Board

- Able to submit proof satisfactory to the Board, substantiated by proper affidavits, of completion of an approved internship

5 – c

Pharmacists must keep valid records, receipts, and certifications of continuing pharmacy education programs completed for three (3) years and submit the certification to the Board on request.

A pharmacist must complete a minimum of one and five-tenths (1.5) CEUs (fifteen (15) contact hours) annually between January 1 and December 31.

6 – a

1.5 CEU (or 15 continuing education hours) are required annually from January 1 to December 31. A pharmacist shall:

- Complete a minimum of one and five-tenths (1.5) CEU (fifteen (15) contact hours) annually between January 1 and December 31; and not transfer or apply excess hours or units for future years.

- A pharmacist may be granted a deferral on a year-to-year basis at the discretion of the Board for illness, incapacity, or other extenuating circumstances.

- A pharmacist first licensed by the Board within twelve (12) months immediately preceding the annual renewal date shall be exempt from the continuing pharmacy education provisions for that year.

7 – d

The Board shall establish standards for pharmacist intern certification and an approved internship program shall determine appropriate qualifications for pharmacists supervising approved internship programs. Each internship certificate is valid for 6 years from date of issuance. The fee for a certificate of internship is set by the administrative regulation and is not to exceed fifty dollars ($50).

8 – b

The following are important renewal dates to remember:

- A pharmacist license must be renewed by February 28 of each year.

- A pharmacy permit must be renewed by June 30 of each year.

- A manufacturer permit must be renewed by September 30 of each year.

9 – e

Within thirty (30) days after the renewal period, the executive director must notify all pharmacists who have failed to comply with license renewal requirements.

Any pharmacist who has failed to renew his license for any consecutive period up to five (5) years may renew his license only upon satisfying the continuing education regulations of the Board and paying the cumulative penalty and renewal fees provided for in KRS 315.110.

Any pharmacist who has failed to renew his license for five (5) or more consecutive years may renew his license only upon satisfying the continuing education regulations of the Board, passing a satisfactory examination before the Board and paying the renewal and penalty fees provided for in KRS 315.110.

Any pharmacist not currently holding an active pharmacist's license in another jurisdiction who does not desire to meet the qualifications for active license renewal shall, upon application, be issued an inactive license. Such license shall entitle the license holder to use the term "pharmacist" but the license holder shall not be permitted to engage in the practice of pharmacy.

An inactive license holder may apply for an active license as provided for by the regulations of the Board. The inactive license renewal fee shall be set by administrative regulation of the Board, not to exceed fifty dollars ($50) annually.

10 – d

The request for expungement may be filed no sooner than three years after the date on which the licensee, permit holder, or certificate holder has completed disciplinary sanctions and if the licensee, permit holder, or certificate holder has not been disciplined for any subsequent violation during this period of time.

11 – d

The Board may refuse to issue or renew a license, permit, or certificate, or may suspend, temporarily suspend, revoke, fine, place on probation, reprimand, reasonably restrict, or take any combination of these actions against any licensee, permit holder, or certificate holder for the following reasons:

- Unprofessional or unethical conduct

- Mental or physical incapacity that prevents the licensee, permit holder, or certificate holder from engaging or assisting in the practice of pharmacy or the wholesale distribution or manufacturing of drugs with reasonable skill, competence, and safety to the public

- Being convicted of, or entering an "Alford" plea or plea of nolo contendere to, irrespective of an order granting probation or suspending imposition of any sentence imposed following the conviction or entry of such plea, one (1) or more for the following, if in accordance with KRS Chapter 335B:
  - A crime as defined in KRS 335B.010
  - A violation of the pharmacy or drug laws, rules, or administrative regulations of this state, any other state, or the federal government

- Knowing or having reason to know that a pharmacist, pharmacist intern, or pharmacy technician is incapable of engaging or assisting in the practice of pharmacy with reasonable skill, competence, and safety to the public and failing to report any relevant information to the Board

- Knowingly making or causing to be made any false, fraudulent, or forged statement or misrepresentation of a material fact in securing issuance or renewal of a license, permit, or certificate

- Engaging in fraud in connection with the practice of pharmacy or the wholesale distribution or manufacturing of drugs

- Engaging in or aiding and abetting an individual to engage or assist in the practice of pharmacy without a license or falsely using the title of "pharmacist," "pharmacist intern," "pharmacy technician," or other term which might imply that the individual is a pharmacist, pharmacist intern, or pharmacy technician

- Being found by the Board to be in violation of any provision of this chapter, KRS Chapter 217, KRS Chapter 218A, or the administrative regulations promulgated pursuant to these chapters

- Violation of any order issued by the Board to comply with any applicable law or administrative regulation

- Knowing or having reason to know that a pharmacist, pharmacist intern, or pharmacy technician has engaged in or aided and abetted the unlawful distribution of legend medications, and failing to report any relevant information to the Board

- Failure to notify the Board within fourteen (14) days of a change in one's home address.

12 – e

The PRNC shall be comprised of eleven members. The members shall include the President of the Board of Pharmacy, the Chair of the PRNC, the Executive Director of the Board of Pharmacy, and eight other members, of which seven must be pharmacists and one must be a citizen member.

13 – b

According to Kentucky pharmacy law, not more than a 4-ounce (120 mL) OTC preparation containing codeine can be dispensed to a single customer within a 48-hour period.

14 – d

The Board shall establish a pharmacist recovery network committee to promote the early identification, intervention, treatment, and rehabilitation of pharmacists and pharmacist interns who may be impaired by reason of illness, alcohol or drug abuse, or as a result of any other physical or mental condition.

15 – e

All decisions revoking or suspending a license, permit, or certificate or placing a licensee, permit holder, or certificate holder on probation or imposing a fine shall be made by the Board. The Board may, when in its opinion the continued practice of the licensee or certificate holder or the continued operation of the permit holder would be dangerous to the health, welfare, and safety of the general public, issue an emergency order as provided in KRS 13B.125.

The Board may, without benefit of a hearing, temporarily suspend a license, certificate, or permit for not more than sixty days if the president of the Board finds on the basis of reasonable evidence that a licensee, certificate holder, or permit holder:

- Has violated a statute or administrative regulation the Board is empowered to enforce, and continued practice or operation by the licensee, certificate holder, or permit holder would create imminent risk of harm to the public.

- Suffers a mental or physical condition that through continued practice or operation could create an imminent risk of harm to the public.

16 – a, b, d
Effective April 1, 2009, a person shall not assist in the practice of pharmacy unless he or she is duly registered as a pharmacy technician under the provisions of this chapter or is exempt under subsection 2.

Subsection 2: A person may assist in the practice of pharmacy without obtaining the registration required by this section if the person:

- Has filed an application with the Board in accordance with KRS 315.136 and no more than thirty (30) days has elapsed since the date the applicant was first employed by the pharmacy. The exemption shall not apply if the application has been denied, the person is less than sixteen years of age, or the person has previously been denied a registration or has had a registration revoked or suspended in any jurisdiction and the registration has not yet been issued or reinstated;

- Is in the employ of a son, daughter, spouse, parent, or legal guardian; or

- Is participating in a work-study program through an accredited secondary or postsecondary educational institution.

17 – b, c, e
Every applicant for registration as a pharmacy technician must be sixteen years of age and of good mental health and moral character and must file with the Board an application in such form and containing such data as the Board may reasonably require.

The application fee shall be twenty-five dollars ($25). Any applicant who serves as a pharmacy technician on a voluntary basis in a pharmacy operated by a charitable provider shall not be required to pay the application fee.

The Board shall issue a certificate of registration and a pocket registration card to an applicant who meets the requirements for registration.

18 – d
Members will serve a term, which is defined as four years. Members can be reappointed once for a total of eight years of service to the Board throughout their lifetime. No member may be appointed to serve more than two full terms.

19 – e
Every pharmacy technician must keep his or her current certificate of registration conspicuously displayed in the technician's primary place of employment.

In addition to a current certificate of registration, each pharmacy technician shall be issued, upon renewal, a pocket registration card which shall be in the registrant's possession when the registrant is assisting in the practice of pharmacy. The pocket registration card shall be exhibited upon the request of any member, inspector, or agent of the Board.

There is no requirement to have continuing education in order to practice as a pharmacy technician in Kentucky. Each technician's registration expires annually on March 31.

Every pharmacy technician who wishes to renew his or her registration shall pay to the executive director of the Board an annual renewal fee of twenty-five dollars ($25) and shall file with the Board an application in such form and containing such information that the Board reasonably determines necessary to renew the registration.

A delinquent renewal penalty fee not to exceed twenty-five dollars ($25) may be assessed for each renewal period the registrant fails to remove his or her registration after the expiration of the registration.

20 – d

Of the six members on the Board of pharmacy, five are required to be pharmacists and one is a citizen at large who is not associated with or financially interested in the practice of pharmacy. No two pharmacists can be from the same county. All members must be residents of the state of Kentucky and in good standing with the Board.

21 – a

When a pharmacist receives a prescription for a brand name drug which is not listed by generic name in the nonequivalent drug product formulary prepared by the Board, the pharmacist must select a lower-priced therapeutically equivalent drug which the pharmacist has in stock, unless otherwise instructed by the patient at the point of purchase or by the patient's practitioner. If a lower-priced selection is made, the label on the container of the drug must show the name of the drug dispensed.

When a pharmacist receives a prescription for a brand name biological product which is not listed by name in the nonequivalent drug product formulary prepared by the Board, the pharmacist must dispense a lower-priced interchangeable biological product, if there is one in stock, unless otherwise instructed by the patient at the point of purchase or by the patient's prescribing practitioner. If an interchangeable product is selected, the label on the container must show the name of the biological product dispensed.

When an equivalent drug product or interchangeable biological product is dispensed in lieu of a brand name drug prescribed, the price of the equivalent drug or interchangeable biological product dispensed must be lower in price to the purchaser than the drug product prescribed.

If, in the opinion of a practitioner, it is to the best interest of the practitioner's patient that an equivalent drug or interchangeable biological product should not be dispensed, the practitioner may indicate in the manner of his or her choice on the prescription "Do Not Substitute," except that the indication must not be preprinted on a prescription.

The selection of any drug or interchangeable biological product by a pharmacist under the provisions of this section must not constitute the practice of medicine.

A pharmacist who selects an equivalent drug product or interchangeable biological product pursuant to KRS 217.815 to 217.826 assumes no greater liability for selecting the dispensed drug product than would be incurred in dispensing a prescription for a drug product or biological product prescribed by its generic, nonbrand, or proper name.

When a pharmacist receives a generically written prescription for a multiple source drug product, he or she must dispense an equivalent drug product in accordance with the provisions of KRS 217.815 to 217.826.

22 – c
The Kentucky State Board of Pharmacy is required to meet at least four times a year. Four members constitute a quorum.

23 – a
The governor appoints the six members of the state Board of Pharmacy. Prior to the end of a member's term, the association will select and submit to the Governor a list of five pharmacists, each of whom has at least five years' experience practicing pharmacy, who is a resident of the state and in good standing with the Board, for the Governor to choose and appoint to fulfill the upcoming vacancy.

24 – e
The Governor may remove a Board member for any of the following reasons:

- Refusal or inability of a Board member to perform his duties as a member of the Board in an efficient, responsible and professional manner;

- Misuse of the office by a member of the Board to obtain personal, pecuniary, or material gain or advantage for himself or another;

- Willful violation of any provision of KRS Chapter 315 or any rule or regulation promulgated thereunder

In the event a Board member is removed, his removal will be effective as of the date of the Governor's finding and a vacancy will be deemed to exist. Any Board member so removed will be entitled to appeal the removal in the Franklin Circuit Court.

25 – b

Continuing education hours shall be approved if approved by the Accreditation Council for Pharmacy Education (ACPE) or the Board.

26 – a, b, e

An automated pharmacy system is a mechanical system that delivers prescribed over-the-counter and legend drugs, and controlled substances received from a pharmacy licensed in Kentucky that maintains transaction information.

Residential hospice facility means a facility that provides residential skilled nursing care, pain management, and treatment for acute and chronic conditions for terminally ill patients.

A pharmacy may provide pharmacy services to a residential hospice facility through the use of an automated pharmacy system under the supervision of a licensed pharmacist pursuant to the policies, procedures, and protocol established by the Kentucky Board of Pharmacy.

The supervising pharmacist must NOT be required to be physically present at the location of the automated pharmacy system and supervision may be provided electronically.

Drugs stored in bulk or unit dose in an automated pharmacy system in a residential hospice facility must be considered the inventory of the pharmacy providing services to the facility and drugs delivered through the automated pharmacy system must be considered dispensed by the pharmacy.

The Kentucky Board of Pharmacy can promulgate administrative regulations including: accuracy of automated pharmacy system, security of the system, recordkeeping, inventory management, labeling requirements, and training of authorized users.

27– b

Charitable pharmacies must comply with all pharmacy permit requirements except those specifically exempted by the Board. Charitable pharmacies may petition the Board in writing to be exempted from those pharmacy permit requirements that do not pertain to the operation of that charitable pharmacy.

Charitable pharmacies may only dispense prescription legend drug samples or prescription legend drugs to qualified indigent patients of the pharmacy, defined as a patient that has been screened and approved by the charitable organization as meeting the organization's mission of providing pharmaceutical care to those who are without sufficient funds to obtain legend drugs.

The charitable pharmacy should NOT charge any fee for the dispensing of prescription legend drug samples or prescription legend drugs to qualified indigent patients.

A charitable pharmacy may accept legend drugs in their unbroken original packaging from pharmacies, wholesalers, or manufacturers, provided appropriate records of receipt and dispensing are maintained. A charitable pharmacy may NOT accept or dispense controlled substances.

28 – b
A pharmacy shall be allowed to place drugs with a home health agency's authorized employees and with a hospice's authorized employees for the betterment of public health. The pharmacy shall remain the legal owner of the drugs.

A written agreement between the pharmacy and home health agency or hospice shall document the protocol for the handling and storage of the drugs by authorized employees and shall be approved by the pharmacist in charge.

The following legend drugs shall be allowed under these agreements:

- Sterile water for injection or irrigation

- Sterile saline solution for injection or irrigation

- Heparin flush solution

- Diphenhydramine injectable

- Epinephrine injectable

- Glucagon

- Influenza vaccine

- Pneumonia vaccine.

29 – a
A pharmacist must complete a minimum of 1.5 CEU (continuing education units), which is equivalent to 15 contact hours annually.

30 – a, c, d
The report should include the following at a minimum, if known and applicable:

- Name, national drug code, and quantity of each controlled substance involved

- A description of the circumstances of the loss

- Names and contact information of witnesses

- Name and description of any person suspected of committing the offense or causing the loss

The Board of Pharmacy may by administrative regulation authorize a pharmacy to submit a completed DEA 106 form in lieu of this data.

31 – c, d, e

Returns or exchanges of prescriptions drugs may or may not be salable according to Kentucky Revised Statutes, 315.404. Drug products may be returned to the original manufacturer, a third-party returns processor, or a reverse distributor licensed as a wholesale distributor.

A wholesale distributor may receive prescription drug returns or exchanges from a pharmacy, pharmacy warehouse, or other person authorized to distribute a prescription drug to an end user under the terms and conditions of an agreement between the parties.

Manufacturers and wholesalers that supply prescription drugs must do so only to a person or entity licensed to possess or distribute prescription drugs to an end user. The prescription drugs supplies by a manufacturer or wholesale distributor shall be delivered only to the business address of the licensee or the address listed on the license.

A licensed wholesaler, pharmacy, or other person authorized to furnish prescription drugs to an end user shall be accountable for their returns process and shall ensure all aspects of operations are secure and do not permit the entry of adulterated or counterfeit prescription drugs.

32 – e

An expungement means that the affected records shall be sealed, the proceedings to which they refer shall be deemed not to have occurred and the affected party may properly represent that no record exists regarding the matter expunged.

The following violations are considered to be minor in nature:

- Failure to renew a license or permit in a timely manner

- Failure to obtain required CE in a timely manner

- Failure to obtain required HIV/AIDS CE in a timely manner

A pharmacist seeking expungement of a record of disciplinary action resulting from the above subsections shall NOT have been the subject of a subsequent violation of the same nature for three years after the date of completion of disciplinary sanctions imposed for the violations sought to be expunged. They should also submit a written request to the Board requesting expungement. The Board considers each request and, if the conditions above are satisfied, expunge every record relating to the subject disciplinary order.

33 – a, c, d

A pharmacist-in-charge is responsible for quality assurance programs, procurement, storage, security, and disposition of drugs, assuring that all pharmacists and interns employed by the pharmacy are currently licensed, providing notification in writing within 14 days of any change in the employment of the pharmacist-in-charge, employment of staff pharmacists, or schedule of hours for the pharmacy.

The pharmacist-in-charge should be designated on the application for a permit to operate a pharmacy, should serve as the PIC for only one pharmacy at a time unless written approval is obtained by the Board, and must be present at the pharmacy at least 10 hours per week to provide supervision.

34 – a

No person may operate a pharmacy within this Commonwealth, physically or by means of the Internet, facsimile, phone, mail, or any other means, without having first obtained a permit as provided for in KRS Chapter 315. An application for a permit to operate a pharmacy must be made to the Board upon forms provided by it and must contain such information as the Board requires, which may include affirmative evidence of ability to comply with such reasonable standards and rules and regulations as may be prescribed by the Board. Each application must be accompanied by a reasonable permit fee to be set by administrative regulation promulgated by the Board pursuant to KRS Chapter 13A, not to exceed two hundred fifty dollars ($250).

Upon receipt of an application of a permit to operate a pharmacy, accompanied by the permit fee not to exceed two hundred fifty dollars ($250), the Board shall issue a permit if the pharmacy meets the standards and requirements of KRS Chapter 315 and the rules and regulations of the Board. The Board shall refuse to renew any permit to operate unless the pharmacy meets the standards and requirements of KRS Chapter 315 and the rules and regulations of the Board. The Board shall act upon an application for a permit to operate within thirty (30) days after the receipt thereof; provided, however, that the Board may issue a temporary permit to operate in any instance where it considers additional time necessary for investigation and consideration before taking final action upon the application. In such event, the temporary permit shall be valid for a period of thirty (30) days, unless extended.

A separate permit to operate is required for each pharmacy.

Each permit to operate a pharmacy, unless sooner suspended or revoked, shall expire on June 30 following its date of issuance and be renewable annually thereafter upon proper application accompanied by such reasonable renewal fee as may be set by administrative regulation of the Board, not to exceed two hundred fifty dollars ($250) nor to increase more than twenty-five dollars ($25) per year. An additional fee not to exceed the annual renewal fee may be assessed and set by administrative regulation as a delinquent renewal penalty for failure to renew by June 30 of each year.

35 – a, b, c, d

A preceptor must be actively engaged in the practice of pharmacy in the location where the pharmacist intern performs his or her internship. The preceptor must supervise only one (1) pharmacist intern at a time for the purpose of the intern obtaining credit for the practice of pharmacy experience, unless the pharmacist is supervising interns as a faculty member at a school or college pharmacy approved by the Board during an academic experience program.. All of the other statements are true.

36 – c

Certified pharmacy technicians under general supervision of a pharmacist can do all of the following:

- Certify for delivery transport systems refilled by another technician.

- Receive diagnostic orders within a nuclear pharmacy.

- Initiate and/or receive a telephone communication from a provider or the provider's agent concerning refill authorization, after identifying themselves as a certified pharmacy technician.

The certified pharmacy technician may NOT receive verbal or telephone prescription orders from a provider or provider's agent.

37 – e

The pharmacist-in-charge of a pharmacy utilizing an automated pharmacy system shall be responsible for:

- Validation of system accuracy prior to use for distribution to patients

- Ensuring the system is properly maintained, is in good working order, accurately dispenses the correct strength, dosage form, and quantity of drug prescribed, and complies with the recordkeeping, access, and security safeguards pursuant to all applicable state and federal laws

- Assuring medications are reviewed prior to loading into an automated pharmacy system and distribution

- Implementing an ongoing quality assurance program that monitors performance of the pharmacy compounding robotics, which is evidenced by written policies and procedures and requires a continued documented validation of doses distributed on a routine basis and annual review of the quality assurance program

- Establishing policies and procedures if there is a system failure of an automated pharmacy system

- Providing the Board with prior written notice of installation or removal of an automated pharmacy system

- Oversight for assigning, discontinuing, or changing personnel access to the system, including establishment of written policies and procedures for security and control

- Reviewing personnel access on at least an annual basis

- Assuring that the decentralized automated pharmacy system stock is checked at least monthly in accordance with established policies and procedures

The security and/or functioning of hardware and software programming is NOT cared for by institutional IT personnel.

38 – e
The following documentation relating to an automated pharmacy dispensing system must be maintained in the pharmacy:

- The name and address of the pharmacy or inpatient health care facility where the system is being used

- The automated pharmacy system manufacturer's name, model, serial number, and software version

- A description of how the system is used

- Written quality assurance procedures and accompanying documentation of use to determine continued appropriate use of the system

- Written policies and procedures for system operation, access, safety, security, accuracy, emergency medication access, and malfunction which includes clearly defined down time and procedures.

39 – d

The transfer of prescription information for any noncontrolled substance prescription for the purpose of new or refill dispensing may occur if it is orally communicated directly between two (2) pharmacists or pharmacist interns in the Commonwealth or between a pharmacist and an individual located in a state or U.S. Territory or District outside the Commonwealth and similarly credentialed as a pharmacist by that state or U.S. Territory or District.

40 – b

A pharmacy generated profile should be maintained separate from the prescription file. The patient profile should be maintained under control of the pharmacist-in-charge for a period of two years following the last dispensing activity. A medication administration record (MAR) as a part of the institutional record should be retained for a period of 5 years from the date of patient discharge from the facility, or in the case of a minor, the MAR should be maintained for a period of 3 years after the patient reaches the age of majority under state law, whichever is longer.

41 – b, c, e, f

Each compounded preparation dispensed to patients shall be labeled with the following information:

- Name, address, and telephone number of the licensed pharmacy (if product leaves the premises)

- Date

- Identifying prescription number

- Name of each drug, strength, and amount

- Directions for use, including infusion rate

- Required controlled substances transfer warnings

- Beyond use date

- Identity of dispensing pharmacist

- Storage requirements, when applicable

- Auxiliary labels, when applicable

42 – a

The PRNC shall be comprised of eleven members. The members shall include the President of the Board of Pharmacy, the Chair of the PRNC, the Executive Director of the Board of Pharmacy, and eight other members, of which seven shall be pharmacists and one shall be a citizen member.

The Board shall establish a pharmacist recovery network committee to promote the early identification, intervention, treatment, and rehabilitation of pharmacists and pharmacist interns who may be impaired by reason of illness, alcohol or drug abuse, or as a result of any other physical or mental condition.

All records and proceedings of the committee that pertain or refer to a pharmacist or pharmacist intern who is or may be impaired shall be privileged and confidential, used by the committee and its members only in the exercise of the proper function of the committee, not be considered public records, and not be subject to court subpoena, discovery, or introduction as evidence in any civil, criminal, or administrative proceedings, except as described in subsection (8) of this section (below):

The committee may only disclose the information relative to an impaired pharmacist or pharmacist intern if:

- It is essential to disclose the information to persons or organizations needing the information in order to address the intervention, treatment, or rehabilitation needs of the impaired pharmacist or pharmacist intern.

- The release is authorized in writing by the impaired pharmacist or pharmacist intern.

43 – c

The Kentucky Board of Pharmacy has addressed generic labeling and has approved these alternatives when product selection is utilized. Alternatives the Board recognizes in lieu of using just the name of the drug dispensed on the label of the prescription container when product selection [substitution] is made are as follows:

(1) Prasugrel "generic substitution made for" Effient

(2) Prasugrel "dispensed in place of" Effient

(3) Prasugrel "substituted for" Effient

(4) Prasugrel "dispensed for" Effient

(5) Prasugrel "generic as" Effient

44 – b

Labeling and packaging of medications used for outpatients must meet the requirements of state and federal law. All of the other statements are true.

45 –a, b, d, e

In the Commonwealth of Kentucky, the transferring pharmacist must record the following information:

- That the prescription is void

- The name and address of the pharmacy to which it was transferred and the name of the pharmacist receiving the prescription information

- The date of the transfer and the name of the pharmacist transferring the information.

46 – b, c, d

The pharmacist receiving the transferred prescription must record the following information:

- The prescription is a transfer

- Date of issuance of original prescription

- Refill authorization of original prescription (how many refills prescription had upon issuance)

- Date of original dispensing

- Refill authorization remaining and date of last refill

- Pharmacy name and address and original prescription number from which the prescription was transferred

- Name of transferring pharmacist

47 – a

A drug shall be classified as misbranded if:

- Its labeling is false or misleading in any particular way.

- It is in a package form, unless it bears a label containing:

- the name and place of business of the manufacturer, packer, or distributor; and
- an accurate statement of the quantity of the contents in terms of weight, measure, or numerical count.

- Any word, statement, or other information required by or under authority of this Act to appear on the label or labeling is not prominently placed thereon with such conspicuousness (as compared with other words, statements, designs, or devices, in the labeling) and in such terms as to render it likely to be read and understood by the ordinary individual under customary conditions of purchase and use.

- It is a drug and its container is so made, formed, or filled as to be misleading; or

- It is an imitation of another drug; or

- It is offered for sale under the name of another drug.

- It is dangerous to health when used in the dosage or manner; or with the frequency or duration prescribed, recommended, or suggested in the labeling thereof.

- It is a color additive the intended use of which is for the purpose of coloring only, unless its packaging and labeling are in conformity with such packaging and labeling requirements applicable to such color additive.

- It was manufactured, prepared, propagated, compounded, or processed in an establishment in any State not duly registered under section 510 of FDCA.

48 – d
In case of an emergency situation, a pharmacist may dispense a drug listed in Schedule II upon receiving oral authorization of a prescribing practitioner, provided that:

- The quantity prescribed and dispensed is limited to the amount adequate to treat the patient during the emergency period

- The prescription is immediately reduced to writing by the pharmacist and contains all information required except for the signature of the prescribing practitioner

- If the pharmacist does not know the practitioner, they make a reasonable effort to determine that the oral authorization came from a practitioner and good-faith efforts to ensure the prescriber's identity

- Within seven days after authorizing an emergency oral prescription, the prescribing practitioner sends a written prescription for the emergency quantity prescribed to be delivered to the dispensing pharmacist. The prescription shall have written on its face "Authorization for Emergency Dispensing" and the date of the oral order. The written prescription may be delivered to the pharmacist in person or by mail postmarked within the seven-day period, or transmitted as an electronic prescription in accordance with federal law and regulation to include annotation of the electronic prescription with the original authorization and date of the oral order. Upon receipt, the dispensing pharmacist shall attach the paper prescription to the oral emergency prescription which had earlier been reduced to writing.

49 – e

If a pharmacist receives a request for a prescription refill with no refill authorized and the pharmacist is unable to readily obtain refill authorization from the prescriber, the pharmacist may dispense a one-time emergency refill of up to a 72-hour supply of the medication when:

- The prescription refill is not for a controlled substance

- The medication is essential to the maintenance of life or to the continuation of therapy in chronic conditions

- In the pharmacist's professional judgment, the interruption of therapy might reasonably produce undesirable health consequences or may be detrimental to the patient's welfare and cause physical or mental discomfort

- The pharmacist notes on the prescription record the date, the quantity dispensed, and his name or initials

- The emergency refill is followed by authorization from the prescriber for continued therapy

50 – a, b, c, d, e

A physician shall terminate the use of Schedule III or IV amphetamine-like controlled substances if:

- The patient does not demonstrate weight loss and does not attempt to comply with exercise and dietary changes

- The body mass index of the patient without a co-morbid condition is less than twenty-seven (27) and the percentage of body fat is normal at less than thirty (30) percent in females or less than twenty-five (25) percent in males

- The body mass index of the patient with a co-morbid condition is less than twenty-five (25) and the percentage of body fat is normal at less than thirty (30) percent in females or less than twenty-five (25) percent in males

- The patient has regained the weight lost, using sympathomimetics as part of a complete program and reuse of the medication does not produce loss of the weight gain to help maintain a minimum of five (5) percent weight loss

- The patient has obtained a Schedule III or IV amphetamine-like controlled substance from another physician without the prescriber's knowledge and consent.

51 – c

The pharmacist must offer to counsel a patient on matters which he believes will optimize drug therapy with each patient or caregiver:

- Upon the presentation of an original prescription order

- On refill prescriptions, as professional discretion dictates

The offer must be made by the pharmacist in a face-to-face communication with the patient or caregiver, unless, in the professional judgment of the pharmacist, it is deemed impractical or inappropriate.

If deemed impractical or inappropriate, the offer to counsel may be made:

- By the pharmacist designee

- In written communication

- By telephone through access to a telephone service that is toll-free for long distance calls, unless the primary patient population is accessible through a local, measured, or toll-free exchange

- In another manner determined by the pharmacist to be appropriate

Patient counseling must be:

- In person when practical

- With reasonable effort, by telephone

52 – c

The Board of Pharmacy may set time and place for examinations, approve colleges of pharmacy, promulgate administrative regulations pertaining to pharmacists, interns, technicians, pharmacies, wholesale distributors and manufacturers, issue subpoenas, schedule and conduct hearings, issue and renew licenses, investigate complaints or violations of the state pharmacy laws, seize any drug or device found by the Board to constitute imminent danger, and employ an executive director.

The executive director MUST be a pharmacist. The executive director is NOT considered a member of the Board.

53 – d

A pharmacist shall offer counseling to a patient on matters that they believe optimize drug therapy. The offer can be made by the pharmacist face-to-face, in written communication, by telephone or by the pharmacist designee. Patient counseling should include the following elements that the pharmacist has deemed appropriate:

- The name and description of the drug or device.

- Dosage form, dosage, route of administration, and duration of drug therapy.

- Special directions and precautions for preparation, administration, and use by the patient.

- Common severe side or adverse effects or interactions and therapeutic contraindications that may occur with the therapy.

- Techniques for self-monitoring of drug therapy.

- Proper storage of medication.

- Refill information.

- Action to be taken in the event of a missed dose.

54 – b

A patient record system shall, with the exercise of professional judgment, be maintained by a pharmacy for patients for whom prescriptive drug orders are dispensed at that pharmacy location.

A pharmacist, with the exercise of professional judgment, shall establish a procedure for obtaining, recording, and maintaining information required for a patient record.

A pharmacist, or his designee, shall obtain, record, and maintain the information for a patient record.

A patient record must:

- Be readily retrievable by manual or electronic means;

- Enable the pharmacist to identify previously dispensed drugs and known disease conditions;

- Enable the pharmacist to determine the impact of previously dispensed drugs and known disease conditions upon the newly submitted prescriptive drug order; and

- Be maintained for not less than 180 days from the date of the last entry.

A patient record must include:

- Full name of patient for whom the drug is intended;

- Address and telephone number of the patient;

- Patient's age or date of birth;

- Patient's gender;

- A list of all prescriptions obtained by the patient at that pharmacy location for the past twelve (12) months by:
  o Prescription number;
  o Name and strength of medication;
  o Quantity;
  o Date received;
  o Identity of prescriber; and
  o Comments or other information as may be relevant to the specific patient or drug; and

- Individual medical history if significant, including known disease states, known allergies, idiosyncrasies, reactions, or conditions relating to prospective drug use and drug regimen reviews.

55 – c, d, e
A prospective drug use review shall be conducted by a pharmacist prior to dispensing. It shall include an assessment of a patient's drug therapy and the prescription order. A

prospective drug use review shall include a review by the pharmacist of the following:

- Known allergies;

- Rationale for use;

- Proper dose, route of administration, and directions;

- Synergism with currently employed modalities;

- Interaction or adverse reaction with applicable:
  o Drugs;
  o Foods; or
  o Known disease states;

- Proper utilization for optimum therapeutic outcomes;

- Therapeutic duplication;

- Incorrect dosage and duration of treatment;

- Clinical misuse or abuse.

56 a, c, c

Each nuclear pharmacy must be equipped with at least the following items of equipment: Dose calibrator, refrigerator; drawing station, well scintillation counter, microscope, chromatographic apparatus or comparable means of effectively assuring tagging efficiency, portable radiation survey meter; and any other equipment deemed necessary for radiopharmaceutical quality assurance for products compounded or dispensed as shall be determined by the Radiation Control Branch, Cabinet for Human Resources, and the Kentucky Board of Pharmacy.

The immediate outer container (shield) of a radioactive drug to be dispensed must be labeled with the: standard radiation symbol, words "caution radioactive material", radionuclide, chemical form, amount of radioactive material contained in millicuries or microcuries, volume in cubic centimeters (if liquid), requested calibration time for the radioactivity contained, name/address/telephone number of the nuclear pharmacy, prescription number, date, and space for patient's name.

Nuclear pharmacies must maintain records of acquisition and disposition of all radioactive drugs in accordance with administrative regulations of the Radiation Control Branch of the Cabinet for Human Resources.

A nuclear pharmacy CAN receive an oral prescription for a radiopharmaceutical, and must immediately have the prescription reduced to writing or recorded in a data processing system.

Nuclear pharmacies are exempt from general space requirements for pharmacies but must have adequate space, be separate from the pharmacy areas for nonradioactive drugs, be inaccessible to all unauthorized personnel and have a radioactive storage and decay area.

57 – b
A collaborative care agreement must:

- Be in writing

- Be signed and dated by each practitioner and each pharmacist who is a party to it

- Provide the method for referral of patients to be managed under the agreement

- State the method for termination of the agreement

Documentation relating to the care and course of therapy of the patient pursuant to the agreement shall be documented in the patient's record maintained by the pharmacist, provided to the collaborating practitioner, and be readily available to other healthcare professionals providing care to the patient.

A collaborative care agreement, and information and records required by the provisions of this administrative regulation, shall be maintained at the pharmacist's practice site and for at least five years after termination of the agreement.

The terms of the collaborative care agreements (medication initiation, discontinuation, dose titration, laboratory monitoring, etc.) are set forth by the participating parties and are not commented on within the written law.

58 – e
Each nuclear pharmacy must have on the premises current editions or revisions of the following reference materials:

- United States Pharmacopeia-National Formulary with supplements

- State statutes and administrative regulations relating to pharmacy

- State and federal regulations governing the use of applicable radioactive materials

- Text relating to the practice of nuclear pharmacy and radiation safety

59 – e

The central refill pharmacy is defined as a pharmacy located in the Commonwealth that provides packaging, labeling and delivery of a refill prescription product to another pharmacy in the Commonwealth for the purpose of the refilling of a valid prescription.

The central refill pharmacy must either have a written contract with the pharmacy, which has custody of the original prescription authorization for refill dispensing, or be under common ownership with that pharmacy.

The central refill pharmacy must:

- Prepare the label for the refill prescription product, which clearly identifies the name and address of the pharmacy preparing the product for refill dispensing and the name and address of the pharmacy that will receive the prepared product for dispensing to the patient

- In addition to its obligation to maintain complete and accurate records of drug products received and otherwise disposed of, maintain accurate records of the preparation of the refilled prescription product, including the name of the:
  - o Pharmacist who verified the accuracy of the refilled prescription product
  - o Pharmacy preparing the refilled prescription product
  - o Pharmacy to which the prepared refill prescription product is delivered

- Provide the originating pharmacy with written information that describes how a patient may contact the central refill pharmacy if the patient has any questions about the preparation of the prescription refill

- Be responsible for ensuring that the order has been properly prepared and verified by a pharmacist.

The pharmacy to which a prepared prescription refill product is delivered must:

- In addition to its obligation to maintain complete and accurate records of drug products received and otherwise disposed of, maintain complete and accurate records of the receipt and dispensing of the centrally refilled prescription product, including the name of the:
  - o Pharmacist who verified the accuracy of the refilled prescription product prior to its dispensing
  - o Pharmacy preparing the refilled prescription product

- Be responsible for ensuring that the refill has been properly prepared, packaged and labeled

- Provide the patient with written information that described how a patient may contact either:
  - The central refill pharmacy if the patient has any questions about the preparation of the prescription refill
  - The dispensing pharmacy if the patient has any questions about the use of the medication

- Be responsible for adherence to the requirements of 201 KAR 2:210.

60 – b
The one-time transfer of the original prescription information for a controlled substance listed in Schedules III, IV, or V, if any authorized refills remain, for the purpose of dispensing is permissible between pharmacies within six (6) months from the date the prescription was issued.

However, pharmacies electronically sharing a real-time, online database may transfer up to the maximum refills permitted by law and the prescriber's authorization.

61 – e
No legend drug or supplies needed to administer a legend drug that are donated for use may be resold.

62 – a
A pharmacist may dispense a therapeutic equivalent drug product if:

- The ordering practitioner has indicated formulary compliance approval on the prescription, either by writing or by checking a formulary compliance approval box on a preprinted form

- The formulary change is a consequence of the patient's third-party insurance plan

- The product designated as preferred by the third party is in the same therapeutic class as the prescribed drug

The pharmacist must notify the ordering practitioner within 24 hours of the formulary compliance substitution either by facsimile or in writing.

63 – a, b, c, d
A pharmacist desiring to dispense Naloxone shall obtain the Naloxone Dispensing Certificate from the Board.
A pharmacist desiring to achieve certification to initiate the dispensing of naloxone shall complete and submit an Application for Pharmacist Certification for Naloxone Dispensing, Form 1, with the Board and provide the following: name, address, phone

number, pharmacist license number and proof of education and training in the use and dispensing of Naloxone for treatment of opioid overdose.

The Board shall issue the certification to a pharmacist who meets the requirements of this section within thirty (30) days of the receipt of the application.

A physician-approved protocol authorizing a pharmacist to initiate the dispensing of Naloxone should contain:

- Criteria for identifying persons eligible to receive Naloxone under the protocol

- Naloxone products authorized to be dispensed (name, dose, route of administration)

- Education to be provided to the person to whom the Naloxone is dispensed

- Procedures for documentation of Naloxone dispensing

- Length of time the protocol is in effect

- Date and signature of physician approving the protocol

- Name and work addresses of pharmacists authorized to initiate dispensing under the protocol

64 – e

A pharmacist dispensing naloxone to a person must provide verbal counseling and written educational materials, appropriate to the dosage form of naloxone dispensed, including:

- Risk factors of opioid overdose

- Strategies to prevent opioid overdose

- Signs of opioid overdose

- Steps in responding to an overdose

- Information on naloxone

- Procedures for administering naloxone

- Proper storage and expiration of naloxone product dispensed

65 – a, b, c, d, e

"Practitioner" is defined as a medical or osteopathic physician, dentist, chiropodist, or veterinarian who is licensed under the professional licensing laws of Kentucky to prescribe and administer drugs and devices. Practitioners include optometrists, advanced practice registered nurses, or physician assistants when administering or prescribing pharmaceutical agents authorized under their own respective laws.

66 – b

No person engaged in sales at retail shall display hypodermic syringes or needles in any portion of the place of business which is open or accessible to the public. Every person engaged in sales of hypodermic syringes or needles at retail shall maintain a bound record in which shall be kept:

- The name and address of the purchaser

- The quantity of syringes or needles purchased

- The date of the sale

- Planned use of such syringes or needles

The record book must be maintained for a period of two (2) years from the date of the sale and shall be available for inspection during business hours by any law enforcement officer, agent or employee of the Cabinet for Health and Family Services or Board of Pharmacy engaged in the enforcement of KRS Chapter 218A.

No person shall present false identification or give a false or fictitious name or address in obtaining or attempting to obtain any hypodermic syringe or needle.

No person engaged in the retail sale of hypodermic syringes or needles shall:

- Fail to keep the records required by this section

- Fraudulently alter any record required to be kept by this section

- Destroy, before the time period required by this section has elapsed, any record required to be kept by this section

- Sell, or otherwise dispose of, any hypodermic syringe to any person who does not present the identification required by this section

- Disclose the names in said book except to those required by this section.

67 – b

Every manufacturer, distributor, wholesaler, repacker, practitioner, pharmacist, or other person authorized to possess controlled substances shall take an inventory of all controlled substances in his possession at least every two (2) years.

A substance which is added to any schedule of controlled substances and which was not previously listed in any schedule shall be initially inventoried within thirty (30) days of the effective date of the statute or administrative regulation which adds the substance to the provisions of this chapter.

68 – a, b, e

The Drug Addiction Treatment Act allows qualified physicians to treat opioid addiction. They must obtain registration with the DEA, granting them a separate DEA number that begins with an "X", indicating their qualification to treat opioid addiction. Both DEA numbers should be on prescriptions written by qualified physicians.

As of 2016, physicians may see up to 275 patients at their practice site and may prescribe CII (methadone)-CV (various naloxone/buprenorphine combination products).

69 – c

A pharmacy located within the Commonwealth that received a pharmacy permit is required to maintain at least one reference from each of the following categories: pharmacology, drug interactions, drug product composition, and state and federal laws and regulations. Electronic references are acceptable if the information is readily retrievable.

The following is deemed minimum equipment required of a pharmacy:

- A prescription balance with a sensitivity not less than that of a Class 3 balance

- Weights—metric or apothecary—a complete set

- Graduates capable of accurately measuring from 1 mL to 250 mL

- Mortars and pestles—glass, porcelain, or wedgewood

- Spatulas—steel and nonmetallic

- Filtration funnel with filter papers

- A heating unit

- Suitable refrigeration unit for proper storage of drugs

- Ointment slab or ointment papers

A pharmacy may be granted an exemption to required reference material and prescription equipment for the prime purpose of dispensing prescriptions.

70 – c

If a pharmacist receives a request for a prescription refill with no refill authorized and the pharmacist is unable to readily obtain refill authorization from the prescriber, the pharmacist may dispense a one-time emergency refill of up to a 72-hour supply of the medication when:

- The prescription refill is not for a controlled substance

- The medication is essential to the maintenance of life or to the continuation of therapy in chronic conditions

- In the pharmacist's professional judgment, the interruption of therapy might reasonably produce undesirable health consequences or may be detrimental to the patient's welfare and cause physical or mental discomfort,

- The pharmacist notes on the prescription record the date, the quantity dispensed, and his name or initials

- The emergency refill is followed by authorization from the prescriber for continued therapy

71 – b

APRNs can prescribe a 72-hour supply of a schedule II medication, except hydrocodone-containing products, unless they are nationally certified in psych or mental health. If the APRN is certified as a psych/mental health provider, they can write for a 30-day supply of a psychostimulant at a time. APRNs can prescribe hydrocodone combination products in a 30-day supply with no refills. APRNs can prescribe schedule III medications in a 30-day supply without refills as well. APRNs must be entered into a collaborative care agreement with a physician licensed in Kentucky in order to prescribe any scheduled II–V medication. APRNs can prescribe 30-day supplies of CIII–CV prescriptions without refills.

72 – e

The Kentucky Controlled Substances Act considers the following criteria for designation of a drug to be a controlled substance: actual or relative potential for abuse, state of current scientific knowledge, risk to public health, immediate precursor to a controlled substance, and history and current pattern of abuse.

The Act outlines the following criteria for scheduled controlled substances:

- C-I
    - High potential for abuse
    - No accepted medical use

- C-II
    - High potential for abuse
    - Accepted medical use
    - Abuse may lead to severe dependence

- C-III
    - Potential for abuse less than C-I or C-II
    - Accepted medical use
    - Abuse may lead to moderate to low physical or high psychological dependence

- C-IV
    - Low potential for abuse relative to C-III
    - Accepted medical use
    - Abuse may lead to limited physical or psychological dependence relative to C-III

- C-V
    - Accepted medical use
    - Low potential for abuse relative to C-IV
    - Abuse may lead to limited physical/psychological dependence relative to C-IV

73 – e

A written prescription for a Schedule II controlled substance written for a patient in a long-term care facility (LTCF) or for a patient with a documented terminal illness may be dispensed in partial quantities, including but not limited to individual dosage units if:

- The pharmacist records on the face of the prescription whether the patient is "terminally ill" or an "LTCF patient"

- The pharmacist records on the back of the written prescription or on another appropriate record, uniformly maintained and readily retrievable, the following:
    - The date of the partial dispensing
    - The quantity dispensed
    - The remaining quantity authorized to be dispensed
    - The identification of the dispensing pharmacist

- The pharmacist contacts the practitioner prior to dispensing the partial quantity if there is any question whether the patient is terminally ill, since both the pharmacist and the prescribing practitioner have a corresponding responsibility to assure that the controlled substance is for a terminally ill patient

- The total quantity dispensed in all partial dispensing does not exceed the quantity prescribed (meaning the prescription can be filled in multiple smaller portions as long as the partial fills remain within the original units prescribed).

- No dispensing occurs beyond sixty (60) days from date of issuance of the prescription

74 – c

Regarding schedule II controlled substances, a pharmacist may never change or add:

- The patient's name

- The name of the controlled substance (except generic substitution permitted by state law)

- Signature of the practitioner

75 – c

In Kentucky, a pharmacist should not dispense any (non-controlled) drug or device if the prescription is presented more than 365 days after the date of issuance.

Schedule III through V controlled substances must not be dispensed after 180 days from the date of issuance.

Schedule II controlled substances must not be dispensed after 60 days from the date of issuance. A prescription shall not be issued for a practitioner to obtain a controlled substance for the purpose of general dispensing or administering to patients.

76 – c

Every practitioner who is authorized to administer or professionally use controlled substances, must keep a record of substances received by him, and a record of all substances administered, dispensed, or professionally used by him otherwise than by prescription. All of these records must be kept for a period of five (5) years.

Manufacturers and wholesalers must keep records of all controlled substances compounded, mixed, cultivated, grown, or by any other process produced or prepared, and of all controlled substances received and disposed of by them. Every such record must be kept for a period of two (2) years.

Pharmacists must keep records of all controlled substances received and disposed of by them. Every such record must be kept for a period of five (5) years.

77 – e
Prescriptions for Schedule III and IV drugs should not be filled after six months from the date of issue, or refilled more than 5 times within a 6-month period.

78 – e
A prescription for a Schedule II controlled substance may normally be transmitted by the practitioner or the practitioner's agent to a pharmacy via fax, provided the original written and signed prescription is presented to the pharmacist for review before the dispensing of the controlled substance. Under federal law there are three exceptions in which the fax can serve as the original:

- A Schedule II narcotic to be compounded for direct patient administration via parenteral, intravenous, intramuscular, subcutaneous, or intra-spinal infusion route

- A Schedule II narcotic for a patient under hospice care (state or federal program)

- Any Scheduled II substance for a resident of a long-term care facility

Kentucky closely follows federal law. The practitioner must note on the prescription that the patient is in hospice care, if that is the case and the file is maintained like all other prescriptions. A new Kentucky provision passed and is to be implemented January 1st, 2021, states prescriptions for Schedule II drugs must be transmitted electronically with some exceptions.

Additionally, a pharmacist who receives a written, oral, or faxed prescription is not required to verify with the prescriber that the prescription falls under such exceptions. Thus, pharmacists may continue to dispense medications from valid written, oral, or faxed prescriptions.

79 – c
When a patient brings in a new prescription for a CS, the Social Security number of the patient must be obtained.

If the patient does not have a Social Security number, then the driver's license number of the patient must be obtained. If the patient does not have a Social Security number or a driver's license number, then the following can be entered: 000-00-0000.

If the prescription is for an animal, you must enter 000-00-000. If the prescription is for a child who does not have a Social Security number or driver's license, then 000-00-0000 must be entered.

80 – b, c

If the prescription is for an animal, the prescription must state the species of animal for which the drug is prescribed and the full name and address of the owner of the animal.

81 – a

All forms of pseudoephedrine must be stored behind the pharmacy counter. A record of each sale must be made documenting the date of the sale, the name, address, date of birth, and photo ID of purchaser, and the amount sold. The purchaser must be 18 years and older. All records must be maintained for 2 years from the date of sale.

Pseudoephedrine limits are as follows:

- 3.6 grams per purchase

- 7.2 grams per month

- 24 grams per year

82 – d

Under KRS, forgery of a prescription is a class D felony on first defense. Any second or subsequent offense is a class C felony.

83 – c, d, e

Nonprescription medicinal preparations that contain in one hundred (100) milliliters, or as a solid or semisolid preparation, in one hundred (100) grams, not more than two hundred (200) milligrams of codeine or its salts may be sold over the counter subject to the following conditions:

- That the medicinal preparation must contain in addition to the codeine in it, some drug or drugs conferring upon its medicinal qualities other than those possessed by the codeine alone.

- That such preparation must be dispensed or sold in good faith as a medicine, and not for the purpose of evading the provisions of this chapter.

- That such preparation must only be sold at retail without a prescription to a person at least eighteen (18) years of age and only by a pharmacist. An employee may complete the actual cash or credit transaction or delivery.

- That such preparations must not be displayed in areas of the pharmacy open to the public.

- That no person may purchase and no pharmacist or practitioner may sell to the same person within a forty-eight (48) hour period more than one hundred twenty (120) milliliters of an exempt codeine preparation. Any person purchasing in excess of this limitation must be deemed to be in illegal possession.

All pharmacists and practitioners must keep a separate exempt codeine registry showing the following:

- Date

- Name of recipient

- Address

- Name of preparation

- Quantity

- Pharmacist's or practitioner's name

84 – d
Medication guides are approved by the Food and Drug Administration (FDA) to educate patients in an effort to help them avoid serious adverse events associated with certain medications. Under the state of Kentucky, medication guides are required to be dispensed with every new prescription as well as refill prescriptions for biologic agents and other common medications, including: some atypical antipsychotics, proton pump inhibitors, bisphosphonates, nonsteroidal anti-inflammatory drugs, psychostimulants, and antidepressants. A complete list of medications that require medication guides can be found on the FDA's website.

85 – a
For a controlled substance prescription drug order to be legal, it must be issued for a legitimate medical purpose by an authorized individual practitioner acting in the usual course of his or her professional practice.

The responsibility for the proper prescribing of controlled substances is upon the prescribing practitioner, but the pharmacist is responsible for the proper filling of the prescription drug order.

A registered physician, dentist, veterinarian, or podiatrist authorized by this state to prescribe controlled substances can issue a prescription for controlled substances only in the usual course of his or her professional practice.

86 – a, b, c

The filing for controlled substances can be done by the following:

Three Separate Files: one file for CII, a second file for III, IV and V, and a third file for non-controlled substances.

Two Separate Files: Under this method the prescriptions for schedule III, IV, and V must be readily retrievable by stamping them with a red "C" or by a computer system. They can then be filed with the CII prescriptions OR the with the non-controlled substances.

There is no requirement to separate OTC product prescriptions.

87 – e

"Home medical equipment" means durable medical equipment which:

- Withstands repeated use

- Is primarily and customarily used to serve a medical purpose

- Is generally not useful to a person in the absence of illness or injury

- Is appropriate for use in the home.

No person shall provide home medical equipment and services, or use the title "home medical equipment and services provider" in connection with his or her profession or business, without a license issued by the Board.

88 – e

Partial filling of a Schedule II CS is permitted for patients who are not terminally ill or a resident of an LTCF. The partial filling must be requested by the patient or the prescribing practitioner, and no additional dispensing may occur beyond 30 days from the date of issuance of the prescription.

This would allow for partial dispensing of a Schedule II CS in two different scenarios in the community pharmacy setting:

(1) the pharmacy is unable to fill the prescription and has 72 hours to complete the filling, or

(2) the patient or prescribing practitioner requests a partial fill and the pharmacist may do so for up to 30 days.

89 – a

A pharmacy may at any time forward controlled substances to DEA-registered reverse distributors who handle the disposal of drugs.

The pharmacist may contact their local DEA Diversion Field Office for an updated list of those reverse distributors in their area. When a pharmacy transfers Schedule II substances to a reverse distributor for destruction, the distributor must issue an Official Order Form (DEA Form-222) to the pharmacy.

When Schedule III–V controlled substances are transferred to a reverse distributor for destruction, the pharmacy should document in writing the drug name, dosage form, strength, quantity and date transferred.

The DEA registered reverse distributor who will destroy the controlled substances is responsible for submitting a DEA Form-41 to the DEA when they have been destroyed.

A DEA Form-41 should not be used to record the transfer of controlled substances between the pharmacy and the registered reverse distributor.

90 – a, b, d, e

For the State of Kentucky, only the following mid-level practitioners can either prescribe, administer, or both prescribe and administer schedule II controlled substances:

- AS (Animal Shelters): Can administer and procure Schedule II and III controlled substances. Line 1 requires Animal Shelter's name and Line 2 requires ET'S Name.

- NP (Nurse Practitioner): Can prescribe Schedule II to V controlled substances (prescribe only).

- OD (Optometrists): Can prescribe and administer Schedule III, IV and V controlled substances. Can prescribe only Schedule II Hydrocodone-containing products.

- Dentists and podiatrists must prescribe within their scope of practice, but do not have restrictions on the prescribing of controlled substances.

PA (Physician's assistant): May not prescribe any Schedule II controlled substance. May prescribe and administer Schedules III, IV, and V controlled substances with limitations.

91 – c

"Special pharmacy permits" means a permit issued to a pharmacy that provides miscellaneous specialized pharmacy service and functions.

"Medical gasses" means oxygen (USP) and nitrous oxide.

The pharmacist-in-charge must review the records of the special pharmacy permit for medical gasses not less than once each quarter. There is no home health aide requirement.

92 – e

During a Governor-issued emergency, if a pharmacist receives a request for a prescription refill with no refill authorized and the pharmacist is unable to readily obtain refill authorization from the prescriber, the pharmacist may dispense an emergency refill of up to a 30-day supply of the medication if:

- The Governor has issued an executive order as authorized by KRS 315.500 for the county where the pharmacy is located

- The pharmacist obtains prescription information from:
    - A prescription label
    - A prescription record within the pharmacy
    - A prescription record from another pharmacy
    - A common database
    - The patient
    - Any other healthcare record

- The prescription refill is not for a controlled substance

- The prescription is for a maintenance medication

- In the pharmacist's professional judgment, the interruption of therapy may produce undesirable consequences or may be detrimental to the patient's welfare and cause physical or mental discomfort

- The pharmacist notes on the prescription record the date, the quantity dispensed, and the pharmacist's name or initials.

93 – e

When the Governor declares a state of emergency pursuant to KRS 39A.100, the Governor may issue an executive order for a period of up to thirty days giving pharmacists emergency authority. The executive order must designate the geographical area to which it applies.

In the executive order, the Governor may vest pharmacists with the authority to:

- Dispense up to a 30-day emergency supply of medication

- Administer immunizations to children pursuant to protocols established by the Centers for Disease Control and Prevention, the National Institutes of Health, or the National Advisory Committee on Immunization Practices or determined to be appropriate by the commissioner of public health or his or her designee

- Temporarily operate a pharmacy in an area not designated on the pharmacy permit

- Dispense drugs as needed to prevent or treat the disease or ailment responsible for the emergency pursuant to protocols established by the Centers for Disease Control and Prevention or the National Institutes of Health or determined to be appropriate by the commissioner of public health or his or her designee to respond to the circumstances causing the emergency.

94 – e
The laminar air flow hood, ISO class 5 environments, ISO class 7 environment and other equipment must be certified annually by an independent contractor in accordance with federal standard 209B and NSF standard No. 49.

95 – e
A confidential record is privileged. A pharmacist may release a confidential record only to:

- The patient or the patient's authorized representative

- A practitioner or another pharmacist if, in the pharmacist's professional judgment, the release is necessary to protect the patient's health and well-being

- The Board or to a person or another state or federal agency authorized by law to receive the confidential record

- A law enforcement agency engaged in investigation of a suspected violation

- A person employed by a state agency that licenses a practitioner, if the person is performing the person's official duties

- An insurance carrier or other third-party payor authorized by the patient to receive the information

96 – d
Records in a Schedule V (OTC) bound book should be maintained for at least 2 years from the date of the last transaction.

97 – a

The following have been determined by the Board to be non-interchangeable unless the United States Food and Drug Administration considers them therapeutically equivalent as published in the "Approved Drug Products with Therapeutic Equivalence Evaluations":

- Digitalis glycosides

- Antiepileptic drugs

- Antiarrhythmic agents

- Conjugated estrogens

- Esterified estrogens

- Warfarin anticoagulants

- Theophylline products

- Thyroid preparations

98 – a, c, d, e

A prescription for a controlled substance must contain the following security features:

A latent, repetitive "void" pattern screened at five (5) % in pantone green must be printed across the entire front of the prescription blank. If a prescription is photocopied, the word "void" must appear in a pattern across the entire front of the prescription;

A watermark must be printed on the backside of the prescription blank so that it can only be seen at a forty-five (45) degree angle. The watermark must consist of the words "Kentucky Security Prescription," and appear horizontally in a step-and-repeated format in five (5) lines on the back of the prescription using twelve (12) point Helvetica bold type style;

An opaque symbol must appear in the upper right-hand corner, one-eighth (1/8) of an inch from the top of the prescription blank and five-sixteenths (5/16) of an inch from the right side of the prescription blank. The symbol must be three-fourths (3/4) of an inch in size and disappear if the prescription copy is lightened;

Six (6) quantity check-off boxes must be printed on the form and the following quantities must appear: 1-24, 25-49, 50-74, 75-100, 101-150, 151 and over

A logo may appear on the prescription blank. The upper left one (1) inch square of the prescription blank must be reserved for a logo;

The following statement must be printed on the bottom of the prescription blank: "Prescription is void if more than one (1) prescription is written per blank"

Refill options must appear below any logo on the left side of the prescription blank in the following order: Refill NR 1 2 3 4 5; and

A prescription blank must be four and one-quarter (4 1/4) inches high and five and one-half (5 1/2) inches wide.

A prescription must bear the preprinted, stamped, typed, or manually printed name, address and telephone number of the prescribing practitioner.

A prescription blank for a controlled substance must NOT contain:

- An advertisement on the front or the back of the prescription blank

- The preprinted name of a controlled substance; or

- The written, typed, or rubber-stamped name of a controlled substance until the prescription blank is signed, dated and issued to a patient.

Only one (1) prescription may be written per prescription blank.

99 – a, b, e
Schedule II amphetamine or amphetamine-like substances can be used to treat the following:

- Narcolepsy

- Attention-deficit/hyperactivity disorder

- Resistant depressive disorder in combination with other antidepressant medications or if antidepressants are contraindicated

- Drug induced brain dysfunction

- Investigational indications with approval from the Board

100 – b

The following are important expiration dates to remember:

- Pharmacy technician registration expires on March 31 of each year.

- A pharmacist license expires on February 28 of each year.

- A pharmacy permit expires June 30 of each year.

- A manufacturer permit expires on September 30 of each year.

Contact Us

Pharmacy Testing Solutions is committed to publishing high-quality, accurate test prep materials. We have had multiple pharmacists review this material as well as a copyeditor. However, despite our best efforts, we realize that an occasional error may occur. If you encounter anything that appears to be incorrect, please contact us!

We will immediately review the issue and publish a correction if necessary. This will help to ensure that our content is 100% accurate for future students. And we will also send you a nice reward for any significant errors that are brought to our attention. You may contact us at: PharmacyTestingSolutions@gmail.com.

Thanks for choosing our MPJE review book!

Made in the USA
Monee, IL
07 July 2023